JANSSEN
PHARMACEUTICAL LIMITED

Grove, Wantage, Oxon OX12 0DQ. Telephone Wantage (023 57) 2966. Telex 837301

With Compliments

Anaesthetists Information Service

Aspects of Recovery
from Anaesthesia

Aspects of Recovery from Anaesthesia

Edited by

Ian Hindmarch
Human Psychopharmacology Research Unit,
University of Leeds

J. Gareth Jones
Anaesthetic Department,
University of Leeds

and

Edward Moss
Anaesthetic Department,
Leeds General Infirmary

A Wiley Medical Publication

JOHN WILEY & SONS
Chichester · New York · Brisbane · Toronto · Singapore

Library of Congress Cataloging in Publication Data:

Aspects of recovery from anaesthesia/edited by Ian Hindmarch, J.
  Gareth Jones, and Edward Moss.
    p.   cm—(A Wiley medical publication)
  Includes index.
  ISBN 0 471 91819 9
    1. Anesthetics—Physiological effect—Congresses. 2. Anesthetics—
  Psychological aspects—Congresses. 3 Postoperative period—
  Congresses. 4. Surgery, Outpatient—Congresses. I. Hindmarch,
  I. (Ian), 1944–   . II. Jones, J. Gareth. III. Moss, Edward.
  IV. Series.
    [DNLM: 1. Anesthesiology—congresses. 2. Postoperative Period—
  congresses. WO 200 A838]
  RD82.A75 1987
  617′.96—dc19
  DNLM/DLC
  for Library of Congress   87-29471
                                                                  CIP

British Library Cataloguing in Publication Data:

Aspects of recovery from anaesthesia
  1. Anaesthesia
  I. Hindmarch, I.   II. Jones, J. Gareth
  III. Moss, Edward
  617′.96   RD81
  ISBN 0 471 91819 9

Typeset by Acorn Bookwork, Salisbury, Wiltshire.
Printed in Great Britain by St Edmundsbury Press, Bury St Edmunds

Contents

Contributing Authors

J. Z. BHATTI   *Human Psychopharmacology Research Unit, Department of Psychology, University of Leeds, Leeds*

B. J. BRITTON   *John Radcliffe Hospital, Headington, Oxford*

J. W. DUNDEE   *The Queen's University of Belfast, Belfast, Northern Ireland*

R. S. EDMONSON   *The General Infirmary, Leeds*

T. E. J. HEALY   *University of Manchester, U.H.S.M., Manchester*

M. HERBERT   *Behavioural Sciences Section, Department of Psychiatry, Nottingham University Medical School, Nottingham*

I. HINDMARCH   *Human Psychopharmacology Research Unit, Department of Psychology, University of Leeds, Leeds*

M. B. HOOPER   *The General Infirmary, Leeds*

J. G. JONES   *University of Leeds, Leeds*

B. KAY   *University of Manchester, U.H.S.M., Manchester*

C. G. MALE   *University of Keele, Stoke-on-Trent*

R. MARKS   *York District Hospital, York*

K. MILLAR   *Behavioural Sciences Group, Medical Faculty, University of Glasgow, Glasgow*

E. MOSS   *The General Infirmary, Leeds*

J. NOBLE   *The General Infirmary, Leeds*

T. W. OGG   *Day Surgery Unit, New Addenbrooke's Hospital, Cambridge*

A. J. PAIN   *Human Psychopharmacology Research Unit, The University of Leeds, Leeds*

P. S. SEBEL   *London Hospital Medical College, Whitechapel, London*

Participants in the Discussion

I. M. BALI *Waveney Hospital, Ballymena*

V. D. BRIM *The General Hospital, Temeside*

P. GOULDEN *Staincliffe General Hospital, Dewsbury*

J. GREENAM *The District General Hospital, Scarborough*

D. R. HAINES *Royal Infirmary, Hull*

S. A. HARGRAVE *Royal Victoria Hospital, Newcastle upon Tyne*

HAW *Pinderfields General Hospital, Wakefield*

HEGGIE *Royal Victoria Hospital, Newcastle upon Tyne*

T. JACK *The General Infirmary, Leeds*

M. KANE *Luton and Dunstable Hospital, Luton*

W. A. McGOWAN *Londonderry, Northern Ireland*

A. McHUTCHON *Queen Elizabeth Hospital, Tyne and Wear*

S. MADSON *Royal Alexandra Infirmary, Paisley*

J. MILLAR *The Churchill Hospital, Oxford*

K. MILLIGAN *Queen's University Hospital, Belfast*

E. PARBROOK *University of Glasgow, Glasgow*

J. E. ROBINSON *The Royal Infirmary, Chester*

C. SMITH *The London Hospital, London*

H. SPEEDY *St Thomas Hospital, London*

S. SRIVASTAVA *South Shields General Hospital, South Shields*

P. M. THORPE *The General Hospital, Kidderminster*

Preface

Efficient, economical and effective day case surgery places demands on surgeons, hospital administrators, nursing staff and anaesthetists. There are also demands made on the anaesthetic induction agents and analgesics used in such relatively short operative procedures. The duration of anaesthesia and/or the postoperative residual effects of anaesthetics should be controlled and limited to the time span of the patient's short stay in hospital. Residual anaesthetic activity in ambulant patients after discharge from hospital could well interfere with the activities of everyday living including risk-prone activities such as operating industrial machinery or driving motor vehicles.

The fact that psychological performance and higher cognitive functions, such as memory and attention, might be impaired following short-term anaesthetic procedures has led to demands on psychologists and psychopharmacologists to develop reliable and valid measures by which possible residual effects might be assessed in the day case patient.

An effective assessment of the residual effects of anaesthesia requires the close co-operation and collaboration of physicians, surgeons, psychologists, pharmacologists and anaesthetists. Short acting anaesthetics and the technology of their administration have to be coupled with surgical operations of similar duration. The psychological effects of such interventions have to be assessed to see at what time—postoperatively—a patient is fit, not just physically, to return to normal daily activities where demands are made on performance, memory and cognitive function. The following papers were presented at a conference which developed out of the co-operation between the Department of Anaesthesia, Leeds General Infirmary and the Human Psychopharmacology Research Unit, University of Leeds. The initial collaborative study, carried out in Leeds General Infirmary, owes much to the initiative and inspiration of the late Professor Gordon McDowall. The editors remember with gratitude Gordon McDowall's contribution to anaesthesia not only in Leeds but also in national and international arenas.

We thank the authors who wrote chapters for the book, and those who contributed to the discussion periods at the conference; these have been edited and included in this volume. We are grateful to George Beaumont for recording and editing the discussion periods, and to the Medical Department of Janssen Pharmaceutical (UK) Ltd, for their kind encouragement and support of the meeting.

Ian Hindmarch
J. Gareth Jones
Edward Moss

Aspects of Recovery from Anaesthesia
Edited by I. Hindmarch, J. G. Jones and E. Moss
© 1987 John Wiley & Sons Ltd

1

A Surgeon's View of Day Case Surgery

B. J. Britton

John Radcliffe Hospital, Oxford

Introduction

For the past 150 years most surgical practice has been based on the principle that recovery from an operation requires rest in a hospital bed. In times past, complications were common and the relief of pain required skilled nursing care. Nowadays the morbidity of most operations is very low and adequate pain relief is easily provided with tablets. General living standards are good and in the UK there is a comprehensive community health care service led by general practitioners. All this means that recovery from many minor and intermediate operations can take place safely in the patient's own home. Patients certainly prefer this and so does the Government. The shorter the hospital stay the less the cost per case and so the more cost-effective the Health Service. However, the day case approach does represent a substantial change in surgical practice and if day case surgery is to be successful it requires careful attention to the following details.

Selection

Choosing the right patient

It is important to pick the right patient for day care. People who can easily appreciate what is involved and accept the idea with enthusiasm are ideal. Some patients are frightened by the responsibility day care entails. They should be offered admission. Children are particularly suitable for day care and up to half of all paediatric surgery can be done on a day case basis (Atwell, 1978). The elderly and the infirm are usually unsuitable and so are the obese because surgery is more difficult and the complication rate is high. For similar reasons, patients with a significant medical condition such as insulin dependent diabetes or a cardiac pacemaker are usually unsuitable.

After their operation, we prefer patients to arrange for a relative or friend to take them home rather than use the ambulance service. It should not take longer than half an hour to arrive home and someone must be there and able to stay with the patient at least until he is able to look after himself. Any help needed should be easily administered by a relative and it is important to check that the helper is him or herself fit and mobile. Easy access to a telephone to summon help if problems arise is also important.

The general practitioner must also be happy to look after the patient at home. His co-operation will be easier to achieve if he knows that immediate help and re-admission will be unquestionably forthcoming if problems do arise. Most of these criteria can be relaxed for minor operations under local anaesthesia, e.g. excision of sebaceous cyst.

Finally, patients must be given a free choice. Most of them know they will have to wait longer for in-patient treatment. Some of them will prefer to do so.

The operation

Approximately two million operations are performed each year in England and Wales and at least one third of them come into the minor and intermediate category and so are potentially suitable for day care (Table 1). Endoscopic and orthopaedic procedures are omitted from the list and, allowing for the fact that only a proportion of the patients will be suitable, it still means that perhaps a quarter or a fifth of all surgery could be done on a day case basis.

Selecting suitable operations

The criteria for selecting suitable procedures for day care can be separated into those that matter before, during or after the operation. Most branches of surgery have some operations which are suitable.

Table 1. Number of operations performed each year in England and Wales. From *Hospital In-Patient Enquiry*, 1976, 1977. Corrected to the nearest 10 000

Dilatation and curettage	130 000
Legal abortion	130 000
Tonsillectomy and adenoidectomy	100 000
Herniorrhaphy	90 000
Cystoscopy	80 000
Operations on the skin	60 000
Anal operations	60 000
Circumcision, orchidopexy, vasectomy	40 000
Surgery for varicose veins	30 000
Total	720 000

Before surgery

The diagnosis must be reliable. Circumcision and termination of pregnancy are straightforward but it may not be appropriate to remove a mole as a day case if there is a chance that it is a malignant melanoma.

Similarly, a lymph node biopsy often appears easy but such nodes may lie close to or even infiltrate vascular structures and so their removal can be haemorrhagic and difficult. On the other hand, it makes no difference whether a groin hernia is indirect or direct, inguinal or femoral. The surgeon can easily adapt the operation to suit the findings and still send the patient home the same day.

Procedures which require special pre-operative preparation in hospital are unsuitable although bowel preparation at home is usually adequate for most anal procedures.

During surgery

The operation should be simple and relatively short. The Royal College of Surgeons in its *Guidelines for Day Case Surgery* (1985) suggest a maximum of 30 minutes general anaesthesia which is quite sufficient for the majority of day case operations. Nevertheless, surgery for varicose veins or an inguinal hernia often takes longer and both are still perfectly acceptable. Operations which open a visceral cavity, with the exception of a hernia, are unsuitable and no drains or tubes should be needed in the wound. However, small suction drains can be inserted for a few hours and removed before the patient goes home. It is also perfectly acceptable to pack an abscess cavity or to leave a plaster cast on a limb for example. Further treatment can easily be arranged either with the district nurse or in the outpatient department.

After surgery

The first requirement is that patients must be able to drink and possibly eat by the time they leave hospital. Similarly, any drugs that are necessary must be available in an oral form. The patient should also be reasonably mobile so operations on both feet at once are inappropriate. There must be no need for skilled and frequent nursing or surgical care so most intraocular surgery is inappropriate. Nor should regular physiotherapy be required although with hand operations, which are often particularly suitable for day care, the patient can be taught his own exercises to practise at home.

The surgical complication rate must be known to be low and those complications that do occur must not be life-threatening. The risks of a serious arrhythmia or reactionary haemorrhage make inserting a pacemaker or a haemorrhoidectomy too dangerous.

Technique

Anaesthesia

Both local and general anaesthesia can be used for day case patients and the anaesthetist has an essential role to play in selecting the most appropriate technique although the choice may be dictated by the type of surgery that is proposed. Some day case operations, such as endoscopy or minor skin operations under local anaesthesia, are usually carried out without the help of an anaesthetist.

Occasional emergencies arise in these patients and it is important to remember that they have received drugs which may affect their recovery.

General anaesthesia

General anaesthesia for day care demands more professional support and a greater degree of vigilance than local anaesthesia. There may be minor operations but there is never a minor general anaesthetic. Experienced anaesthetists and recovery staff are essential. The ease of operating under such conditions may also encourage the surgeon to embark on procedures which are too extensive for day care. Such patients must be admitted at least overnight.

Local anaesthesia

Epidural and spinal blocks are the province of the anaesthetist in the developed world and both have a place in day surgery. Regional anaesthesia is well within the scope of the surgeon himself. This saves the anaesthetist's time and does not demand full recovery facilities. Long-acting local anaesthetics (e.g. bupivacaine) provide excellent post-operative pain relief and they can also be used at the end of operations under general anaesthesia. If adrenaline is also used, meticulous haemostasis is essential as there is an increased risk of haematoma formation.

Local anaesthesia does impose some constraints. The anaesthesia must be complete so the surgeon must wait until the block is fully established. No parenteral analgesic short of general anaesthesia will compensate for an inadequate block and since general anaesthesia is very occasionally needed, patients should always be starved beforehand. The operative field is also restricted which may be inconvenient and the operations usually take longer.

Surgical technique

A standard surgical operation must always be done. There can be no question of an inadequate procedure being followed simply because the patient is a day case. Meticulous surgical technique is essential and this will minimize post-operative discomfort and reduce the number of complications. This means sharp dissection where possible, careful haemostasis and, above all, gentle handling of the tissues. Local anaesthesia is particularly valuable at teaching all these points. The smaller the amount of tissue damage, the less likely are post-operative pain and risk of infection. Primary closure of the wound is best if it is possible and subcuticular absorbable sutures are ideal. The wound is then sealed at once and no nursing time is needed for suture removal.

Because surgical skill is very important in successful day care, most people have recommended that only senior staff should undertake day surgery. Younger surgeons must learn, however, and whilst it is not appropriate to begin a surgical career in a day unit, once some experience is gained, trainees can easily undertake day case work. As in all other surgical training, careful case selection and proper supervision is then essential.

Post-operative care

Patients who receive a general anaesthetic need time to recover before going home and they may also need some analgesia before departing. After a local anaesthetic it is best if the patient returns home to bed at once before sensation returns. All the patients will need a supply of analgesic tablets and some may require an antiemetic as well. Analgesia after the operation always raises anxiety in patients' minds, is often difficult to manage and remains a significant problem with day care. Efficacy and absorption of oral analgesics varies widely as does patients' perception of pain. Most people can provide their own minor analgesic such as aspirin or paracetamol but some patients will need and must be given a small supply of oral morphine or pethidine tablets. It is essential that the patient, a relative or friend, fully understands how to use the tablets they are given.

The aim of this type of surgery should be to reduce the demands on the community health care team to a minimum. Nevertheless, some patients will need help from the district nurse. Often this is general advice and moral support but a few patients will need dressings changed or sutures removed. Many patients will be able to come to the Health Centre to have this done.

Organization

Efficient arrangements must be made to ensure that all the usual records, measurements and investigations are completed and the results available in the right place at the right time. Because the patient is only in the hospital for short periods of time, this process must be fast.

Speed in relation to individual patients and the rapid turnover of large numbers of patients inevitably means a greater risk of mistakes. These can only be reduced to an absolute minimum by laying down clearly defined policies for handling patients, their relatives and their records, which are understood and adhered to by all the staff.

At the initial outpatient visit, it must be established and recorded that the patient is socially and medically suitable for day case treatment. This takes extra time which must be allowed for in the outpatient booking times. Any necessary investigations must be ordered. At some stage, suitability for day case anaesthesia must be decided either in outpatients, at a pre-admission anaesthetic outpatient clinic or on the morning of admission. When the patient arrives at the hospital all the admission details must be recorded and medical staff must be available briefly to clerk the patient, to confirm that the right procedure is planned, to check that the discharge arrangements are satisfactory and to obtain written consent if this has not already been done in the outpatient department.

After the operation, all the normal rules for recovery from anaesthesia apply. The relative or friend who will escort the patient home must arrive on time. Any tablets that are needed must be available. Finally, the wound must be checked for excessive bleeding and provided all is well, the patient is escorted or wheeled to his transport.

All of this is very much easier to organize within a designated day case unit, but there is nothing that cannot be organized perfectly satisfactorily in an ordinary surgical ward if necessary.

The final piece of organization which is absolutely essential is that a few in-patient beds must be available to take those patients who unexpectedly are unable to go home. This will happen to between 3 and 5% of patients whose treatment was originally planned on a day case basis (Goulbourne and Ruckley, 1979).

Information

None of these arrangements will work unless the patient and his helper fully understand exactly what is involved and exactly what they will be required to do. Most patients nowadays like to know about their operation but this is more important in day cases. It means explaining the operation in language that is suitable for the individual and it also includes information about apparently mundane matters such as constipation, mobility, analgesic tablets and what to do when things apparently go wrong. All this information must be provided at the first outpatient interview. It can be supplemented with an information sheet or tape cassette which the patient can read or listen to at home. Any queries can be dealt with when the patient comes for surgery.

It is equally important to inform the general practitioner when his patients have had their operations and returned to his care. The surgeon should telephone the practice and follow this up with a letter which the patient can deliver to the surgery on the way home.

If all these points are carefully followed then day case surgery will provide efficient, satisfactory and, above all, safe treatment.

References

Atwell JD (1978) Changing patterns in paediatric surgical care. *Ann. Roy. Coll. Surg. Eng.*, **60**, 375–83.

Goulbourne AA and Ruckley CV (1979) Operations for hernia and varicose veins. *Br. Med. J.*, **2**, 712–14.

Royal College of Surgeons of England (1985) *Guidelines for Day Case Surgery*. London: RCSE.

Aspects of Recovery from Anaesthesia
Edited by I. Hindmarch, J. G. Jones and E. Moss
© 1987 John Wiley & Sons Ltd

2

An Anaesthetist's View of Day Case Surgery

T. W. Ogg

New Addenbrooke's Hospital, Cambridge

The day patient is 'a person attending hospital for *non-resident* investigation, therapeutic tests or operation'. The concept of day surgery is not new but it has become an attractive proposition for District Health Authorities striving to provide a surgical service for the 700 000 patients presently awaiting surgery in England and Wales.

In 1982 the Cambridge Health Authority was faced with shortages of financial resources and nursing staff. Furthermore, the closure of Old Addenbrooke's Hospital resulted in a loss of in-patient surgical beds. A working party under the chairmanship of the author planned and erected a 12 bedded purpose-built day surgery unit at a cost of £300 000 (Ogg, 1985). The unit was opened in 1983 and there are now 10 operating sessions per week. Seven of the surgeons with lists in the unit have also dropped an in-patient operating session. Table 1 shows the main advantages and disadvantages of day case surgery. It is important to stress that day surgery should not be regarded as a second class service but that it should be developed on its own merits.

Work-load of the Cambridge Day Surgery Unit

A total of 8016 minor and intermediate operations were performed in the day surgery unit during 1984–86. The main users were the gynaecologists (48.9% of the total work-load), orthopaedic surgeons (16.5%), urologists (14.6%) and the ENT surgeons (9.7%).

Eighty per cent of all surgery was performed under general anaesthesia and senior surgeons and anaesthetists were involved in the majority of operations. The hospital admission rate for 1984–86 from the day surgery unit was 0.2%. Furthermore, despite a reduction of in-patient beds, the specialities involved

Table 1. Advantages and disadvantages of day-case surgery

Advantages	Disadvantages
Large number of patients treated	Regarded by some surgeons as a second-class service
Fewer nurses required	Good pre-operative selection is essential
Good nurse recruitment	Doubts about the ideal anaesthetic techniques
Psychological benefits (children)	
Reduced surgical waiting lists	Minor sequelae *will* occur after surgery and anaesthesia
Reduced cross-infection rates	Problems of recovery and driving
Economic benefits (dependent on a reduction of in-patient beds)	Possible increase in work-load of the community services

in the day surgery unit have recorded a 19.35% decrease of their in-patient waiting lists. These findings may hasten an expansion of the existing day unit. The East Anglian Regional Health Authority has already estimated that by the year 2000, 25% of all surgery in the region will be performed on a day case basis.

Pre-operative assessment

Outpatients may pose medical problems for the anaesthetist when they attend for day surgery (Ogg, 1976). A simple pre-operative assessment question-naire was devised (Figure 1) and a series of 200 outpatients recorded incidences of cardiovascular, respiratory and metabolic problems, ranging from 42 to 57%. Good anaesthetic practice demands that anaesthetists should assess all patients before anaesthesia to ensure their fitness for surgery. Outpatient anaesthetic assessment clinics have their problems and only the anaesthetist who adminsters the general anaesthetic can realistically assess his own patients. Anaesthetists should be especially wary of orthopaedic patients attending day units. Many of these patients have been waiting 3–5 years for surgery and their medical histories may alter with time. These patients should be invited to complete and return a pre-operative assessment form one month before scheduled surgery. Table 2 shows the pre-operative selection guidelines issued to all surgical firms working in the day unit.

It is most important that pre-operative investigations are kept to an absolute minimum. Finally, experience has shown that the pre-operative guidelines issued may be disregarded so constant vigilance by anaesthetists is required.

Cambridge Health Authority	Surname:	
Addenbrooke's Hospital	First name:	Hospital number:
Day Surgery Unit	Consultant:	Date of birth:
Day Case Form	Department:	Male/female:

To be completed by the patient PLEASE TICK CORRECT ANSWER   YES   NO

Have you had anything to eat or drink in the last 6 hrs?   ...   ...
Will you have to go home alone?   ...   ...
Will you be on your own when you get home?   ...   ...
Will this be your first operation?   ...   ...
Have you had any serious illness?   ...   ...
Have you had any problems with anaesthetics?   ...   ...
Has any of your family had any problems with anaesthetics?   ...   ...
Have you a cough, cold or nose trouble?   ...   ...
Do you get breathlessness or chest pain on exercise or at night?   ...   ...
Do you get swollen ankles?   ...   ...
Have you had heart disease, rheumatic fever or high blood pressure?   ...   ...
Do you have bronchitis, asthma, chest pain or other chest problems?   ...   ...
Do you smoke?   ...   ...
Have you ever had convulsions or fits?   ...   ...
Do you faint easily?   ...   ...
Do you drink a lot of alcohol?   ...   ...
Do you have arthritis or prolonged muscle disease?   ...   ...
Do you have anaemia or other blood problems?   ...   ...
Do you bruise or bleed excessively?   ...   ...
Do you have allergies or reactions to medicines, etc?   ...   ...
Are you on any medicines now? (tablets, capsules, injections, inhalations)   ...   ...
Have you ever been jaundiced?   ...   ...
Have you ever had any urinary or kidney troubles?   ...   ...
Have you ever had diabetes or sugar in the urine?   ...   ...
Are you pregnant?   ...   ...

IT IS DANGEROUS TO DRIVE, RIDE A BICYCLE, OPERATE MACHINERY OR USE A COOKER ON *THE DAY YOU HAVE AN ANAESTHETIC — THANK YOU FOR YOUR HELP*

To be completed by nurse

Weight .... kg   Haemoglobin .... g/dl   LMP ....   B/P ....

Operation planned ....

Consent forms signed?   YES/NO   Loose or artificial teeth present: YES/NO
Jewellery removed?   YES/NO   Identification bracelets?   YES/NO

Multistix: Urobilinogen ....   Blood ....   Bilirubin ....   Ketones ....

Glucose ....   Protein ....   pH ....

Figure 1. Pre-operative assessment form.

Table 2. Cambridge Day Surgery Unit pre-operative selection guidelines

---

- Patients must be accompanied home.
- Age limit of 70 years.
- Patients should live within a 20 mile radius of the unit.
- Patients should be fit and healthy (ASA 1 and 2).
- Please exclude surgical procedures where severe post-operative pain or haemorrhage may occur.
- Exclude patients who are either obese, diabetic or who have chronic respiratory cardiovascular disease.
- No food nor liquids should be taken orally for 6 hours prior to general anaesthesia or local anaesthesia with intravenous sedation.
- Operations should not exceed 30 minutes duration.

---

*Doubts on age and physical fitness should be discussed with the Consultant Anaesthetist in charge of the day surgery unit.

Post-operative assessment

Morbidity

It is now widely recognized that minor post-operative sequelae do occur after a brief general anaesthetic. A study by Ogg in 1972 reported an incidence of drowsiness (26%), headaches (27%), nausea (22%) and dizziness (11%) in a group of 100 day cases attending hospital for urological operations. These sequelae may be significantly reduced by modern general anaesthetic techniques lasting a maximum of 30 minutes. All patients attending the Cambridge Day Surgery Unit are advised before surgery that post-operative side-effects such as nausea and drowsiness may occur. Mothers returning home to young children should also be advised to have responsible help for the first 24 hours after recovery from anaesthesia.

Driving

There is little published evidence to suggest how long the effects of general anaesthetics impair driving skills. It is considered good practice not to allow a patient to drive or ride a bicycle for at least 24 hours following day case anaesthesia (Ogg, 1972). Furthermore any activity which requires skill and judgement should be avoided for 24 hours. Both the patient and the accompanying adult should be informed of these facts.

Recovery

The evaluation of recovery following general anaesthesia is difficult. No single test can adequately demonstrate that patients are free from the influence of an anaesthetic drug and therefore safe to leave hospital.

Anaesthesia for day surgery should ensure a rapid recovery with a swift return to street fitness. It would appear sensible for day cases to regain their ability to respond and to react to environmental stimuli in a conscious, co-ordinated manner in the post-operative period. At Cambridge, a memory function card test is employed to assess recovery from anaesthesia (Ogg *et al.*, 1979) and more recently a computerized visual perception test has been developed (Salt *et al.*, 1985). It appears that general anaesthesia affects the memory recall of *new* facts so caution must be taken when discharging day cases. There is no substitute for the clinical evaluation before patients are discharged from the day surgery unit. Patients should be judged to be alert and orientated, able to tolerate oral fluids, and able to dress and walk unaided. Their vital signs should be stable and they must be accompanied home by a responsible adult. Finally, written and verbal post-operative instructions should be issued, e.g. details of post-operative analgesics prescribed, when to drink, drive and return to work and to contact their own general practitioner in an emergency. Experience to date has revealed that the community medical and nursing services are not overburdened by the Cambridge programme of day surgery. The presence of a community liaison sister in the day unit has done much to smooth the problems arising from early discharge of hospital patients.

The majority of day cases having minor gynaecological operations, e.g. dilatation and curettage and termination of pregnancy are discharged within 2–3 hours of their operation. However, patients having laparoscopies are operated upon first on a morning list and discharged at 1600–1700 hours. Paediatric cases having myringotomies and grommets on an afternoon list may be safely allowed home with their parents approximately one hour following surgery.

Anaesthetic agents suitable for day cases

The ideal day case anaesthetic technique should produce a swift induction, good operating conditions, minimal side-effects and rapid recovery. Most anaesthetists will have their personal preferences but the author's practice is as follows:

Premedication

This is frequently omitted but patients are all reassured by the anaesthetist during their pre-operative visit. Temazepam, the short-acting benzodiazepine, may produce effective anxiolysis with minimal delay of post-operative recovery.

Intravenous anaesthetic induction agents

These should produce a rapid anaesthetic action, pain-free injection, no histamine release, no involuntary movements and rapid recovery. The author has used all the commercially available induction agents and has discarded etomidate and methohexitone because they both produce a high incidence of side-effects.

Propofol has been used for 2000 patients in the Cambridge day unit and is deservedly popular because of rapid patient recovery and lack of sequelae, e.g. vomiting, dizziness and drowsiness. The addition of 1 ml 0.1% lignocaine (plain) to each 20 ml propofol ampoule reduces the incidence of injection site pain. Many anaesthetists continue to use thiopentone for day cases and disregard its hangover effects. Perhaps the time has arrived to test post-operative recovery 24 hours after day case anaesthesia in order to decide whether the cheap, long-acting induction agent (thiopentone) should be used in preference to the more expensive, short-acting agent (propofol).

Anaesthetic supplements

The synthetic, short-acting opiate alfentanil has a definite place in the day unit. Halothane and enflurane remain the popular inhalational agents in the Cambridge day unit. Recently with all the controversy with halothane hepatotoxicity, isoflurane has been used with a closed circuit. Many anaesthetists employ total intravenous anaesthesia for day surgery especially since the introduction of propofol.

Endotracheal intubation

This may be performed safely for both adult and paediatric day cases. However, as a general rule intubation is avoided in the Cambridge day unit but intubation facilities are always close at hand for emergencies. A day case anaesthetic technique for laparoscopy has been developed and patients receive no muscle relaxants, no endotracheal intubation and are allowed to breathe spontaneously (Ogg, 1985). So far, minimal problems have arisen in 1200 laparoscopies and the hospital admission rate is less than 1%.

Other drugs used in the day unit

Local anaesthetic techniques have a definite place in any day unit. They can be used alone, in combination with light general anaesthesia or sedation and for post-operative analgesia. Bupivacaine 0.25% and 0.5% is popular because of its long-lasting effects. Prilocaine 0.5% is used for Biers Blocks and lignocaine 1–2% plain for paracervical blocks.

Finally, all patients anaesthetized in the Cambridge day unit are closely monitored (ECG, blood pressure and pulse).

Conclusion

Day surgery is an attractive proposition for patients, nursing staff and administrators alike. It is only one of the ways open for the NHS to increase its efficiency. The planned programme of day surgery at Cambridge has been a worthwhile, cost-effective exercise which has reduced in-patient surgical waiting lists. Anaesthetists have much to offer in the organization of any day care programme, for patients must be carefully assessed, given adequate pre- and post-operative instructions and, after general anaesthesia, safely returned into the community. There is no doubt that day surgery will expand in Britain over the next decade.

References

Ogg TW (1972) An assessment of post-operative cases. *Br. Med. J.*, **4**, 573–6.
Ogg TW (1976) An assessment of pre-operative cases. *Br. Med. J.*, **1**, 82–3.
Ogg TW (1985) Aspects of day surgery and anaesthesia. *ICU Anaesth. Rounds*, **18**, 1–28.
Ogg TW *et al.* (1979) Day case anaesthesia and memory. *Anaesthesia*, **34**, 784–9.
Salt PJ, Francis RI, Noble J and Ogg TW (1985) Assessment of recovery from anaesthesia using a new visual perception test. *Br. J. Anaesth.*, **57**, 820–21.

Aspects of Recovery from Anaesthesia
Edited by I. Hindmarch, J. G. Jones and E. Moss
© 1987 John Wiley & Sons Ltd

3

Morbidity following Day Case Anaesthesia

E. Moss and M. B. Hooper

The General Infirmary, Leeds

Introduction

Morbidity following day case anaesthesia can be the result of surgery, anaesthesia, or a combination of both. The potential surgical morbidity includes haemorrhage, severe pain, deep venous thrombosis and infection. Deep venous thrombosis is extremely unlikely in a patient who is ambulant immediately before and soon after surgery and patients who are likely to suffer severe post-operative pain should not undergo day case surgery. Careful attention to surgical technique should keep the incidence of post-operative haemorrhage and infection to a minimum.

The potentially serious anaesthetic morbidity includes complications of pre-existing disease (e.g. myocardial infarction and respiratory insufficiency), complications of concurrent drug therapy (e.g. insulin, anticonvulsants and steroids), chest infections, drug reactions, laryngeal oedema and potential hazards of failing to obey instructions (e.g. inhalation of stomach contents and personal accidents). Careful selection of patients will eliminate many of these problems. The use of non-irritant plastic tracheal tubes should reduce the likelihood of laryngeal oedema, and observation of the patient for at least two hours post-operatively will allow the early detection and treatment of drug reactions and airway problems.

The price that has to be paid for the convenience, efficiency and economy of day case surgery is an increased incidence of minor post-anaesthetic sequelae. These include feeling unwell, drowsiness, headache, nausea, vomiting, dizziness, unsteadiness, sore throat and pain (Fahy and Marshall, 1969; Ogg, 1972). In addition, the use of suxamethonium in day cases is associated with a very high incidence of post-operative muscle pains (Churchill-Davidson, 1954) and is probably best avoided (see below). Although some minor sequelae are inevitable, the minor morbidity associated with day case anaesthesia and surgery may be reduced by using local analgesia (Muir, 1976; Ogg *et al*., 1983), developing techniques of general anaesthesia which give fewer sequelae (Ogg *et al*., 1983) and developing better techniques for the relief of pain, for example, the use of local analgesia. Finally, it has been suggested that gradual mobilization and advice to go to bed on arriving home will reduce the occurrence of minor post-operative sequelae (Bali and Kendrick, 1985).

Oral Surgery

Because of an insufficient number of in-patient beds in Leeds, it has been necessary to perform certain oral surgical operations requiring tracheal intubation as day cases. Two studies of post-operative morbidity following day case anaesthesia were carried out in patients undergoing these procedures. In the first study, an attempt was made to find the best method of avoiding suxamethonium pains in day cases. In the second study, the effect of duration of anaesthesia on morbidity following day case relaxant anaesthesia was assessed.

Methods

First study

450 patients undergoing day case tracheal anaesthesia for oral surgical procedures were allocated to one of nine groups. The following anaesthetic agents were administered to supplement in each case nitrous oxide, oxygen and halothane:

Group A—thiopentone, suxamethonium
Group B —methohexitone, suxamethonium
Group C —Althesin, suxamethonium
Group D—propanidid, suxamethonium
Group E —etomidate, suxamethonium
Group F —Gallamine 20 mg (1 minute before the suxamethonium), Althesin
                or etomidate, suxamethonium
Group G—Gallamine 20 mg (3 minutes before the suxamethonium), Althesin or etomidate, suxamethonium
Group H—Althesin or etomidate
Group I —Althesin, fazadinium

Patients in groups A to H breathed spontaneously and in group I were ventilated mechanically. All were intubated with a plastic nasotracheal tube and a pharyngeal pack was inserted. The patients were sent a questionnaire seven days after the operation. The questionnaire asked specifically about muscle pains, sore throat and feeling unwell and had a space for individual comments.

Second study

A further 106 patients were studied in whom anaesthesia was induced with etomidate followed by fentanyl 50 mg, glycopyrrolate 0.2 mg and atracurium 0.4 mg/kg. A plastic nasotracheal tube and gauze pharyngeal pack were inserted and the patients were ventilated mechanically with nitrous oxide, oxygen and halothane 0.5%. At the end of the procedure the muscle relaxant was reversed with neostigmine and atropine. Post-operatively the patients completed two questionnaires, the first approximately two hours after termination of anaesthesia before leaving the day unit, and the second seven days later at the surgical follow-up appointment. The patients were divided into two groups according to the duration of the anaesthesia. Anaesthesia lasted for 30 minutes or less in the first group and more than 30 minutes in the second group.

The Chi-squared test, Student's t-test and Wilcoxon unpaired rank sum test were used as appropriate to compare the different groups.

Results

First study— reduction of post-operative suxamethonium pains

In the first study, 375 patients returned the questionnaire giving an overall reply rate of 83%. The nine groups were comparable with regard to age, weight and sex distribution. The incidence of muscle pains which were severe and/or inconvenienced the patients is shown in Figure 1. In groups A to E, the incidence was approximately 50% with the induction agent having very little influence on the incidence of pains.

Pre-treatment with gallamine 20 mg (groups F and G) reduced the incidence of muscle pains, but increasing the time between administration of the gallamine and the suxamethonium did not produce any further reduction. Groups H and I showed a very low incidence of muscle pains and acted as a control group. When the incidence in the control groups was subtracted from that in groups A to G, the incidence of suxamethonium pains which were severe or inconvenienced the patient was 43% in groups A to E and 22% when patients were pre-treated with gallamine (groups F and G) ($P < 0.001$).

Table 1 compares the incidence of sore throat in patients who had a V-pack inserted in the pharynx with that following a gauze pharyngeal pack. The incidence and duration (which can be taken as an index of severity) of sore throat were similar with both types of pack.

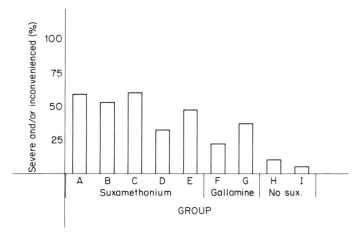

Figure 1. The incidence of muscle pains which were severe and/or inconvenienced the patients.

The incidence of other complaints in this study and a comparison with the results of other workers is given in Table 2. Of our patients, 74% felt abnormal when they left the One Day Unit.

Second study—morbidity and duration of anaesthesia

The overall incidence of complaints was the same in both groups (Table 3). There were one or more complaints from 86% of patients at the time of discharge and 94% after leaving hospital. There was a high incidence of

Table 1. The incidence of sore throat following packing of the pharynx with a gauze pack or a V-pack. Both groups were anaesthetized with etomidate, suxamethonium, nitrous oxide, oxygen and halothane. The gauze pack group were pretreated with gallamine 20 mg

	Gauze pack	V-pack
Number of patients	35	41
Sore throat		
Yes	83%	78%
No	17%	22%
Duration (hours)	57.6	63.6
SD	±41.0	±37.4

Table 2. Incidences of other complaints in this study compared with those in other studies

	This study %	Fahy & Marshall (1969) %	Muir (1976) %	Smith & Young (1976) %	Heneghan et al. (1981) %
Felt abnormal	74	45	—	—	—
Dizzy or lightheaded	39	6	39	51	19
Headache	13	13	27	81	—
Weakness in legs	26	—	—	—	19
Drowsy	8	30	68	73	18
Nausea and vomiting	12	16	34	47	11

feeling unwell (75%), dizziness (67%), unsteadiness (68%), drowsiness (78%), sore throat (80%), and pain at the injection site (20%), but the results of visual linear analogue measurements, employed to assess the severity of some of these complaints, indicated that only about 30% of the patients suffered badly (i.e. marked the 10 cm line at more than 5 cm).

The incidence of nausea was higher after leaving hospital and the incidence

Table 3. Duration of anaesthesia and overall incidence of post-anaesthetic complaints (the number of complaints reported expressed as a percentage of the total number of possible complaints)

	Duration of anaesthesia	
	<30 min	>30 min
Number of patients	59	47
Age		
mean	20.9	25.9
range	12–53	11–52
Sex		
M	9	19
F	50	28
Duration of anaesthesia (min)		
mean	21.9	39.1
range	15–30	31–60
Patients complaining (%)		
2 hours	86	87
7 days	93	95
Overall incidence of complaints (%)		
2 hours	49	46
7 days	41	36

of vomiting was 22%. Dizziness was the only complaint which showed a significant difference in incidence between the two groups ($0.05 > P > 0.02$). The incidence was higher following the shorter anaesthetics. On average, no complaint lasted for more than 48 hours. Concentration was impaired in 20% on leaving the unit but only 8% complained of this problem after they arrived home. About 5% complained that their memories were affected and 16% complained of post-operative cough and/or sputum.

Summary

The first report of the occurrence of muscle pains following the administration of suxamethonium was that of Bourne and colleagues in 1952, and in 1954 Churchill-Davidson demonstrated that the highest incidence of post-suxamethonium pains was in those patients who were ambulant in the early post-operative period particularly in those undergoing anaesthesia as out-patients. Churchill-Davidson found a 66% incidence of muscle pains with a 44% incidence of pains which were severe or incapacitating, which compares well with our figures of 59% and 43% respectively in the suxamethonium groups.

From the suxamethonium groups in our study, the group receiving pro-panidid showed the lowest incidence of muscle pains, and this finding agrees with that of Clarke and his colleagues (1964). However, no anaesthetic induction agent produced a sufficient reduction in the incidence or severity of the muscle pains to recommend its use in preference to the others.

Various methods of reducing post-suxamethonium pains have been sug-gested which include using as small a dose of suxamethonium as possible, giving the suxamethonium by slow infusion (Lamoreaux and Urbach, 1960), pre-treatment with a small dose of suxamethonium (Burtles and Tunstall, 1961), the administration of a small dose of non-depolarizing muscle relaxant at least one minute before the suxamethonium (Churchill-Davidson, 1954; Morris and Dunn, 1957; Lamoreaux and Urbach, 1960; Dottori *et al.*, 1965; Glauber, 1966), the administration of neostigmine after respiration is fully recovered (Foster, 1960) and pre-treatment with lignocaine (Wilkinski *et al.*, 1965). Most of these investigations have been performed on in-patients so their relevance to outpatients is questionable. The results of this study show that pre-treatment with gallamine 20 mg significantly reduced the incidence and severity of muscle pains following suxamethonium, and that no benefit was gained by giving the gallamine more than one minute before the suxa-methonium.

The incidence of sore throat following tracheal anaesthesia is high (Thomp-son, 1975; Baron and Kohlmoos, 1975; Smith and Young, 1976). In this investigation, use of a V-pack (Vickery and Burton, 1977) did not alter the incidence or severity of sore throat.

The majority of patients felt abnormal or unwell when they recovered consciousness. In the first study, only 8% complained of drowsiness, possibly because they expected to feel drowsy after an anaesthetic, and only 12% vomited, an incidence which compares favourably with that in other studies.

Some authors have found that the incidence of minor post-anaesthetic sequelae increases when the operation lasts more than 15–20 minutes (Fahy and Marshall, 1969; Ogg, 1972), and Ogg *et al.* (1983) have recommended that anaesthesia for day case oral surgery should not last for more than 30 minutes. Sometimes oral surgical procedures unexpectedly last longer than 30 minutes, so it is an important finding that the incidence of minor post-anaesthetic sequelae does not increase as the duration of anaesthesia increases when a light anaesthetic using a non-depolarizing muscle relaxant is employed. Such an anaesthetic technique has the additional advantages that the incidence of dysrhythmias is reduced (Miller *et al.*, 1970; Thomas *et al.*, 1976, 1978), suxamethonium pains are avoided and there is a rapid return of protective reflexes. The incidence of vomiting (22%) was high and this may be a disadvantage of the relaxant technique (Heneghan *et al.*, 1981). However, this could probably be reduced by the use of antiemetics.

These studies show that the incidence of minor morbidity after day case tracheal anaesthesia is high, but of short duration. The only way of avoiding suxamethonium pains in day case anaesthesia is to avoid suxamethonium. The use of a non-depolarizing muscle relaxant and light anaesthesia not only avoids suxamethonium pains, but also eliminates the influence of duration of anaesthesia on post-anaesthetic morbidity.

References

Bali IM and Kendrick RW (1985) Alfentanil and isoflurane for day stay dental surgery. *Anaesthesia*, **40**, 702–3.

Baron SH and Kohlmoos HW (1975) Laryngeal sequelae of endotracheal anaesthesia. *Anesth. Analg.*, **54**, 767–8.

Burtles R and Tunstall ME (1961) Suxamethonium chloride and muscle pains. *Brit. J. Anaesth.*, **33**, 24.

Churchill-Davidson HC (1954) Suxamethonium (succinylcholine) chloride and muscle pains. *Br. Med. J.*, **1**, 74.

Clarke RSJ, Dundee JW and Daw RH (1964) Clinical studies of induction agents XI: The influence of some intravenous anaesthetics on the respiratory effects and sequelae of suxamethonium. *Br. J. Anaesth.*, **36**, 307.

Dottori O, Lof BA and Ygge H (1965) Muscle pains after suxamethonium. *Acta Anaesthesiol. Scand.*, **9**, 247–56.

Fahy A and Marshall M (1969) Postanaesthetic morbidity in out-patients. *Br. J. Anaesth.*, **41**, 433–8.

Foster CA (1960) Muscle pains that follow the administration of suxamethonium. *Br. Med. J.*, **2**, 24.

Glauber D (1966) The incidence and severity of muscle pains after suxamethonium when preceded by gallamine. *Br. J. Anaesth.*, **38**, 541–4.

Heneghan C, Macauliff R, Thomas D and Radford P (1981) Morbidity after outpatient anaesthesia. A comparison of two techniques of endotracheal anaesthesia for dental surgery. *Anaesthesia*, **36**, 4–9.

Lamoreaux LF and Urbach KF (1960) Incidence and prevention of muscle pain following administration of succinyl chlorine. *Anesthesiology*, **21**, 394.

Miller JR, Redish CH, Fisch C and Oehler RC (1970) Factors in arrhythmia during dental outpatient general anaesthesia. *Anesth. Analg.*, **49**, 701–6.

Morris DDB and Dunn CH (1957) Suxamethonium chloride administration and post-operative muscle pain. *Br. Med. J.*, **1**, 383.

Muir VMJ, Leonard M and Haddaway E (1976) Morbidity following dental extraction: a comparative survey of local analgesia and general anaesthesia. *Anaesthesia*, **31**, 171–80.

Ogg TW (1972) An assessment of post-operative outpatient cases. *Br. Med. J.*, **4**, 573–6.

Ogg TW, MacDonald IA, Jennings, RA and Morrison CG (1983) Day case dental anaesthesia. Evaluation of three methods of anaesthesia. *Br. Dent. J.*, **155**, 14–17.

Smith BL and Young PN (1976) Day stay anaesthesia. A follow-up of day patients undergoing dental operations under general anaesthesia with tracheal intubation. *Anaesthesia*, **31**, 181–9.

Thomas VJE, Kyriakou KP and Thurlow AC (1978) Cardiac arrhythmias during outpatient dental anaesthesia: A comparison of controlled ventilation with and without halothane. *Br. J. Anaesth.*, **50**, 1243–5.

Thomas VJE, Thomas WJW and Thurlow AC (1976) Cardiac arrhythmia during outpatient dental anaesthesia: the advantages of a controlled ventilation technique. *Br. J. Anaesth.*, **48**, 919–22.

Thompson PW (1975) Day case anaesthesia in the dental hospital. *Proc. R. Soc. Med.*, **68**, 415–6.

Vickery IM and Burton GW (1977) Throat packs for surgery. An improved design based on anatomical measurements. *Anaesthesia*, **32**, 565.

Wilkinski R, Usubiaga BLJ, Usubiaga JE and Wilkinski JA (1965) Prevention of succinylcholine fasciculation with local anaesthetics. *Anesthesiology*, **26**, 3–7.

Aspects of Recovery from Anaesthesia
Edited by I. Hindmarch, J. G. Jones and E. Moss
© 1987 John Wiley & Sons Ltd

4

Outpatient Anaesthesia for Urology

R. Marks

York District Hospital, York

Introduction

The problems associated with anaesthetizing patients for urological proce-dures are rather different from those with most other outpatient surgical procedures. The patients are generally in the second half of life, frequently not in the best of physical condition and most importantly the majority of them require repeated anaesthetics over many years at relatively short intervals. Adding to the pressures for outpatient anaesthesia are the long waiting lists for in-patient admission in many units so that the more patients that can be treated as outpatients, the less the demand on in-patient facilities.

The two largest groups of patients are those with carcinoma of the bladder, some of whom manage all their treatment on an outpatient basis, and the women with recurrent urinary tract infections. Another significant group is patients with interstitial cystitis who are managed by frequent hydrodistension of the bladder and present a similar problem, from an anaesthetic point of view, to the bladder cancer patient. Patient selection is, therefore, under certain pressures and involves discussion with the urologist and, if there is any doubt, must be made after in-patient assessment. The safety of the patient must come first, but the criteria emphasized at York are possibly more flexible than those used in many units and in the 20 years of outpatient anaesthesia in our unit, there have been no untoward accidents.

Age is no barrier and several patients in their 90s undergo regular check cystoscopies. The most important factor is whether or not home support is present, as the technique used produces minimal upset even to the frailest of patients and the type of surgery does not produce much in the way of post-operative problems. What is of prime importance is the effect of the anaesthetic technique on the patient's well-being and not, as is usually measured, the effects of the anaesthetic on physiological variables, assuming

25

that the technique actually chosen has inherent safety and suitability for repeated administration.

The need for frequent general anaesthetics in many urology patients makes them an ideal group for assessing patient satisfaction with the anaesthetic. The problem of repeated halothane anaesthetics on the liver first became a cause for concern about 10 years ago, and the author found that methohexitone, in spite of its drawbacks, was a satisfactory agent for day case anaesthesia. Patients recover from it much more rapidly than from thiopentone, and while there is some evidence that it produces a secondary peak blood level at four hours, in practice this does not seem to be a problem. There is a low incidence of sensitivity reactions to it and premedication is not necessary. Patients are given full written instructions including the advice to avoid alcohol, driving and operating any machinery on the day of the anaesthetic.

Day Case Anaesthesia for Urological Surgery

A simple trial was designed to test patient satisfaction. All the patients entered into the trial had previously been anaesthetized by the author using a methohexitone, nitrous oxide and halothane sequence and were familiar with the unit and the after-effects of endoscopic urology. Two different techniques were compared, the standard one mentioned above and a technique utilizing fentanyl and avoiding halothane. All the anaesthetics were administered by the author and all the operations were performed by the same consultant urologist. The techniques were chosen randomly and the observations made by the same nursing staff who were in ignorance of the technique used.

The patients were all given a questionnaire to fill out at home and post back after each visit. An attempt was also made to assess surgical acceptance of the techniques as a rapid turnover of five to six patients an hour is our usual practice for sessions of 10 to 12 patients. Seventy patients were entered into the trial which took over 18 months to complete. There were 48 male patients, all of whom had carcinoma of the bladder and 22 female patients, four of whom had interstitial cystitis. This made a male to female ratio of 2.67 : 1 for the cancer patients.

The average age of the male patients was 64.6 years and the female patients 65.7, and the average weight of the males was 73.7 kg and the females, 58.2 kg.

The duration of anaesthesia ranged from three to 21 minutes, the halothane group average being 7.2 minutes and the fentanyl group 6.8 minutes.

The halothane anaesthetic consisted of an induction dose of methohexitone 1 mg/kg body weight followed by nitrous oxide and oxygen supplemented by halothane. The fentanyl supplemented anaesthetic consisted of giving a bolus of fentanyl initially, in a dose of 1 μg/kg, followed by methohexitone in the same dose as before and supplemented by nitrous oxide and oxygen with

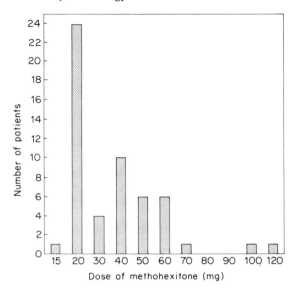

Figure 1. Distribution of incremental doses of methohexitone in the fentanyl group.

additional doses of methohexitone if movement occurred or seemed immi-nent. These additional doses ranged from 20 to 170 mg (Figure 1). None of the patients was premedicated. The distribution of duration of anaesthesia is shown in Figure 2.

Hiccough, coughing, spontaneous muscle movements and respiratory depression were noted. Mild meant that the side-effect stopped before surgery commenced, moderate that it continued for up to two minutes into the operation and severe was longer than that and usually interfered with the operation.

As opiates are frequently advocated to reduce the incidence of hiccoughing due to methohexitone, it was surprising to find an increased incidence in the fentanyl technique. The overall 24.3% in the halothane series is comparable to other published results but the 35.7% in the fentanyl patients is rather high, though most of these fall into the mild category.

Coughing is a significant problem, possibly because many of the patients are bronchitic and still smoke. Of those receiving the halothane anaesthetic 22.9% coughed whereas only one patient coughed after fentanyl.

Spontaneous muscle movements and twitching are difficult to differentiate so they are grouped together. The figure for halothane of 14.3% accords with the usual incidence while fentanyl reduced it by half.

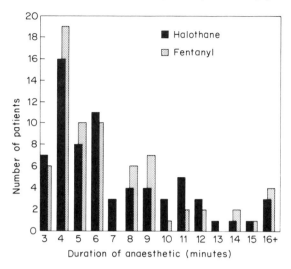

Figure 2. The distribution of duration of anaesthesia.

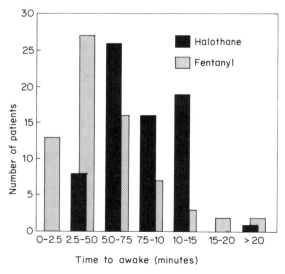

Figure 3. The time taken to awake in the two
anaesthetic groups.

Respiratory depression to a minor degree occurred in five of the fentanyl patients, who required ventilatory assistance for a few breaths—it was not a cause for concern.

Both techniques produced equally satisfactory operating conditions: 90% of the patients were still when surgery commenced and only one patient, who had halothane, caused a delay in the surgery.

Recovery from the anaesthesia was appreciably shorter in the fentanyl series. Patients were asked to repeat their name, where they were and the day and date as an indication of recovery. The average recovery time was 8.16 min with halothane with a range of just over 3 min to 33 min 30 sec, and 5.57 min with fentanyl, the range being 1 to 28 min. The eyes open to awake interval was generally shorter with fentanyl (Figure 3).

It is in the category of post-anaesthetic complications that the most significant differences arose. In the recovery room, similar numbers of patients complained of nausea but five patients vomited after fentanyl and none did after halothane. Four of the halothane patients complained of dizziness but more than twice this number (nine) were dizzy after fentanyl—these were patients other than those who had nausea and vomiting. In all, 15.7% of the halothane patients and 28.6% of the fentanyl patients had complications attributable to anaesthesia while in the recovery room.

Fentanyl was expected to reduce the post-operative discomfort associated with cystoscopy and this proved to be the case. Thirty per cent of patients having halothane anaesthesia had discomfort while only 18.6% of the fentanyl group complained. Fifteen patients had equal discomfort with both agents.

Use of a technique avoiding an inhalational agent could produce some degree of awareness. Three patients with halothane and four patients with fentanyl had dreams and one patient dreamt with both agents. There was no incidence of awareness.

The replies to the questionnaire produced the most salutary reminders of what we can do to our patients. A total of 133 of the 140 were returned—a very high response rate. Halothane scored a 92.3% acceptance as that proportion felt well or just drowsy in the first 24 hours. One patient was nauseated but none was sick. Two complained of feeling unwell and two had a headache. Only 68.6% of the fentanyl patients felt well or drowsy, six complained of nausea and a further seven patients vomited at home on more than one occasion. Eight who did not mention nausea or vomiting complained of feeling ill and one had a headache. One patient who had fentanyl required hospital admission for persistent vomiting and another called out his general practitioner because he felt so unwell.

The patients were not asked which technique they preferred, but 22 patients did express a view—nine opting for halothane and 13 for fentanyl. There was no doubt that those patients who did not have side-effects from fentanyl felt much more alert afterwards.

Currently, the author's only change of technique is to use enflurane in place of halothane, but as a comparison of halothane with enflurane cannot be done for ethical reasons, a consecutive group of 55 patients were studied to see if there were any marked differences to halothane. This group was comparable to the previous patients except that the ratio of males to females was reduced.

The incidence of hiccough was about the same but coughing was reduced in comparison to halothane, as were muscle movements. Operating conditions were the same as was the time taken to recover. There was no incidence of nausea or vomiting, but 16.4% complained of headache and two patients felt slightly dizzy. Post-operative discomfort was increased and two of the patients had dreams.

This trial can obviously be criticized on several counts. Alfentanil has been tried with even more disappointing results than fentanyl. A comparative trial using an antiemetic routinely has not been performed, partly because the results are not as good as when an opiate is totally avoided, but mainly because the author aims for simplicity.

This chapter has demonstrated that patients having repeated short anaesthetics seem to do best with a simple inhalational technique. Certainly in this group of patients, any narcotic produces an unacceptably high incidence of complaints. The patients should be consulted as to the acceptability of the technique. Modern outpatient anaesthesia began with cystoscopy sessions and every year the number of day case anaesthetics increases, putting a tremendous burden on all concerned to provide a safe method of outpatient anaesthesia with minimal upset to the patient's well-being. Many of our patients go back to work the next day, and one plays his trombone the same evening. Thus the anaesthetic technique described above is very suitable for day case urological procedures.

Aspects of Recovery from Anaesthesia
Edited by I. Hindmarch, J. G. Jones and E. Moss
© 1987 John Wiley & Sons Ltd

5

Alfentanil-Supplemented Anaesthesia for Short Surgical Procedures

P. S. Sebel

London Hospital Medical College, London

Alfentanil is a short-acting synthetic opioid analgesic. Rapid recovery occurs after both single and multiple doses (van Leeuwen *et al.*, 1981; Bovill *et al.*, 1982) hence it is considered a suitable agent for short surgical procedures such as in day case patients.

Two studies have been completed at the London Hospital, Whitechapel, with the aim of assessing alfentanil-supplemented anaesthesia and paying particular attention to aspects of post-operative recovery. First, alfentanil-supplemented anaesthesia was compared with fentanyl-supplemented anaesthesia in 80 patients undergoing short gynaecological operations (Patrick *et al.*, 1984). Later alfentanil-supplemented anaesthesia was compared with isoflurane-supplemented anaesthesia in 51 patients scheduled for short urological or gynaecological procedures (Short *et al.*, 1984). The participants were randomly allocated to the study groups as shown in Table 1.

All patients were unpremedicated. The dosages of alfentanil were 5 μg/kg followed by 2.5 μg/kg every 8 min, fentanyl 1 μg/kg then 0.5 μg/kg every 16 min, althesin 50 μl/kg plus 1 ml increments as required, methohexitone 1.5 mg/kg plus 20 mg increments as required. Nitrous oxide 66% was given in certain allocated groups. In study B, when isoflurane was administered, it was given initially at concentrations up to 5% reducing to 1.5–2.0% when anaesthesia was satisfactory.

Frequent measurements of respiratory rate, heart rate and arterial blood pressure were made. Peroperative and post-operative side-effects and complications were noted. Early post-anaesthetic recovery was assessed by measuring the time to opening eyes on command and giving their name and date of birth correctly. Late recovery assessed by checking how long post-operatively it was before the patient could perform the post-box test as

Table 1. Alfentanil-supplemented anaesthesia for short surgical procedures—frequency of side-effects and complications (Number of patients in whom these side-effects occurred)

Groups	n	Age (years)	Peroperative complications				Postoperative complications	
			Coughing	Hiccoughing	Spontaneous movements	Number of patients with apnoeic episodes	Nausea	Vomiting
Study A								
Fentanyl, althesin oxygen	20	28	2	1	19	8	7	4
Fentanyl, methohexitone nitrous oxide, oxygen	20	27	0	3	19	7	12	10
Alfentanil, althesin, oxygen	20	26	0	2	18	11	2	1
Alfentanil, methohexitone nitrous oxide, oxygen	20	25	1	6	16	8	8	5
Study B								
Alfentanil, methohexitone nitrous oxide, oxygen	20	45	0	5	14	14	3	0
Methohexitone, isoflurane oxygen	11	46	8	5	9	10	4	2
Methohexitone, isoflurane nitrous oxide, oxygen	20	43	8	6	8	10	2	1

quickly as he or she had done it pre-operatively (Craig *et al.*, 1982). This test consists of measuring the time taken to post 18 moulded plastic shapes through holes into a post-box, and is considered a valid assessment of motor co-ordination. Also the deletion of 'p's test was done to assess concentration either after the post-box test was completed (Study A) or at 45 minutes post-operatively (Study B). The deletion of 'p's test is the deletion of the letter 'p' from a page of random lower case typed letters, 58 lines long and 38 letters per line (Dixon and Thornton, 1973). The score is the number of lines completed in three minutes minus the number of errors made.

For reasons of clarity, the pertinent results from both studies are condensed together in Tables 1 and 2. The results should only be compared between groups within each study. The demographic data are similar within each study but the patients in study B are generally older than those in study A. The duration of surgery was longer in study A compared to study B. In the second paper, the researchers excluded patients having termination of pregnancy as isoflurane could have increased the blood loss during surgery as a result of its effect on uterine contractility (Munson and Embro, 1977). The exclusion of this group of patients is probably responsible for the difference in age and duration of surgery between the studies.

The cardiorespiratory effects of each anaesthetic were clinically acceptable in all groups, except possibly for the incidence of apnoeic episodes. Within each study, the number of patients having apnoeic episodes was similar between the groups; however, the apnoea occurred early in the introduction of isoflurane to patients and was probably related to its pungency. In the opioid groups the apnoea could occur after every increment, but there was no difference between fentanyl and alfentanil, and no patients in study A required assisted ventilation. The older age of the patients in study B may have been the reason for the slightly higher incidence of apnoea in these patients.

There was a significantly higher incidence of coughing in the isoflurane groups, which was so troublesome that the methohexitone–isoflurane–oxygen anaesthetic technique had to be abandoned after completion of 11 cases.

Hiccoughing was present in some patients in all the groups but was most marked in the groups receiving methohexitone. This complication is most probably related to the use of that induction agent.

It was noted in all groups that some spontaneous movements occurred, but while in the isoflurane groups these movements occurred during the induction period, they occurred throughout surgery in the opioid groups. They were never so serious as to disrupt surgery.

Patients having termination of pregnancy are widely considered to be prone to post-operative nausea and vomiting and this may explain the overall difference in the incidence of nausea and vomiting seen between the two studies.

Table 2. Alfentanil-supplemented anaesthesia for short surgical procedures—
recovery data

Groups	Early tests			Later tests	
	Open eyes (min)	Name (min)	Date of birth (min)	Post-box (min)	Net 'p' score (preop– postop)
Study A					
Fentanyl, althesin, oxygen	9.1	11.2	12.2	41.8	2
Fentanyl, methohexitone					
nitrous oxide, oxygen	5.8	7.2	7.8	46.1	4
Alfentanil, althesin, oxygen	7.2	10.8	12.3	34.0	4
Alfentanil, methohexitone,					
nitrous oxide, oxygen	6.4	7.4	7.9	33.3	3
Study B					
Alfentanil, methohexitone,					
nitrous oxide, oxygen	3.3	4.1	4.3	34.3	4
Methohexitone, isoflurane,					
oxygen	9.2	9.5	9.8	44.3	2
Methohexitone, isoflurane,					
nitrous oxide, oxygen	9.1	9.6	9.6	40.2	2

In study A, the incidence of nausea and vomiting was less in patients
receiving alfentanil compared to the patients receiving fentanyl. There was no
difference between isoflurane and alfentanil as a cause of nausea and vomiting
as can be seen from study B.

Recovery data from the two studies are summarized in Table 2. As noted
above, caution must be exercised when looking at these results but within
each study the demographic and other details are similar.

The assessment of early recovery (opening eyes, correct name and date of
birth) in the first study demonstrated a difference between the induction
agents (althesin and methohexitone) but there was no difference between the
opioids fentanyl and alfentanil. In the second study, the induction agent was
methohexitone in all groups and the main comparison was between alfentanil
and isoflurane. The alfentanil group recovered significantly faster than the
isoflurane groups.

The tests of late recovery show that alfentanil has significant advantages
over fentanyl. The post-box test was completed earlier and although the
deletion of 'p's scores are similar, this test was done earlier in the alfentanil
groups. The alfentanil group in study B had a better result for the post-box
test but this was statistically significant only against the isoflurane–oxygen

group and not when compared against the isoflurane–nitrous oxide–oxygen group.

From the peroperative conditions noted, there is little to choose between either of the opioids, fentanyl or alfentanil. Both cause apnoeic episodes and both allow more patient movements during surgery than is usual with an inhalational technique.

However, the opioid techniques may allow a pollution-free anaesthetic and there is less trouble from coughing and movements at induction of anaesthesia. In cases where inhalational vapours have relative contraindications (such as terminations of pregnancy), opioid techniques as detailed in these studies can be used safely.

The more rapid awakening that takes place with alfentanil-supplemented anaesthesia compared to isoflurane-supplemented anaesthesia may be an advantage if there are poor recovery facilities in the operating theatre or in the day case theatre.

It is open to debate as to how far one can extrapolate the results from bedside tests to indicate street fitness. The results from the tests of later recovery are most likely to indicate how the patients would fare later in the day on their discharge from hospital. In these tests, there is no difference between the alfentanil and the isoflurane–nitrous oxide–oxygen techniques. It is clear, however, that alfentanil techniques offer advantages over fentanyl in that the patients could complete the post-box test earlier post-operatively.

The combination of no premedication, methohexitone induction, and isoflurane-supplemented anaesthesia may appear attractive on paper for promoting rapid recovery from anaesthesia. However, there are disadvantages such as pain on injection, hiccoughing and coughing to overcome. By the same token, the use of a very short-acting opioid such as alfentanil, may appear attractive on paper but this has the disadvantages of causing apnoeic episodes and allowing peroperative patient movements. If rapid recovery is required at the expense of smooth anaesthesia, then these techniques as they stand are suitable. It is quite possible, if necessary, to improve the quality of anaesthesia with minor adaptations to the techniques described here.

Premedication with a short-acting benzodiazepine such as temazepam may reduce the coughing and laryngospasm during the introduction of isoflurane. Lignocaine may be given to reduce the pain of injection from methohexitone, or alternatively thiopentone given to induce anaesthesia which may also allow a smoother introduction of isoflurane, cause less hiccoughing and possibly less spontaneous movements than occurred in these studies.

In conclusion, alfentanil offers significant advantages over fentanyl when rapid recovery from anaesthesia is required. Patients take slightly longer to recover from isoflurane anaesthesia when compared with alfentanil but this difference becomes less significant for the later tests of recovery. Therefore, both isoflurane/nitrous oxide-supplemented anaesthesia and alfentanil-supplemented anaesthesia are satisfactory for short surgical procedures such as would be undertaken in day patients when rapid recovery is required.

References

Bovill JG, Sebel PS, Blackburn CL and Heykant J (1982) The pharmacokinetics of alfentanil (R39209): a new opioid analgesic. *Anesthesiology*, **57**, 439–43.

Craig J, Cooper GM and Sear JW (1982) Recovery from day case anaesthesia. Comparison between methohexitone, Althesin and etomidate. *Br. J. Anaesth.*, **54**, 447–51.

Dixon RA and Thornton JA (1973) Tests of recovery from anaesthesia and sedation: intravenous diazepam in dentistry. *Br. J. Anaesth.*, **45**, 207–15.

Munson ES and Embro WJ (1977) Enflurane, isoflurane and halothane and isolated human uterine muscle. *Anesthesiology*, **46**, 11–14.

Patrick M, Eagar BM, Toft DF and Sebel PS (1984) Alfentanil-supplemented anaesthesia for short procedures: A double-blind comparison with fentanyl. *Br. J. Anaesth.*, **56**, 861–6.

Short SM, Rutherford CF and Sebel PS (1984) A comparison between isoflurane and alfentanil supplemented anaesthesia for short procedures. *Anaesthesia*, **56**, 861–6.

Van Leeuwen L, Deen L and Helmers JH (1981) A comparison of alfentanil and fentanyl in short operations with special reference to their duration of action and postoperative respiratory depression. *Anaesthetist*, **30**, 397–9.

Aspects of Recovery from Anaesthesia
Edited by I. Hindmarch, J. G. Jones and E. Moss
© 1987 John Wiley & Sons Ltd

6

Ventilatory Control during Recovery from Anaesthesia

J. G. Jones

University of Leeds, Leeds

Introduction

Ventilatory control has been studied in a number of contrasting conditions such as rest/exercise, health/disease and more recently, consciousness/unconsciousness. During recovery from anaesthesia not only is there a fluctuating state of consciousness which impairs ventilatory control but also a number of other factors may combine to cause a marked degree of hypoxia. In particular there is an impairment of pulmonary gas exchange which may persist for several days into the post-operative period. This is more marked in upper abdominal or intrathoracic operative procedures although it may occur after any general anaesthetic. Although the mechanism is not fully explained it is more likely to be due to persistent alveolar collapse particularly in dependent parts of the lung. This background of hypoxia, which in itself may be harmless, is exacerbated by the combined effects of anaesthetic and analgesic drugs whose deleterious influence on the control of ventilation is enhanced when the patient falls asleep (Catley *et al.*, 1983, Catley, 1984). Extensive studies have now been reported on the respiratory effects of sleep but studies of sleeping patients in the immediate post-operative period are quite limited.

This chapter first describes the effects of sleep in ventilatory control and this will be followed by a description of the interaction of sleep and opioids in the post-operative period.

Effects of Sleep on Ventilatory Control

Sleep is a complex and multivariable state which has been subdivided on the basis of electroencephalographic (EEG) criteria and rapid eye movement

(REM) into a number of stages (Partridge, 1984). Non-REM sleep is divided into four stages, characterized by progressive slowing and increase in amplitude of EEG waves, as the patient's state changes from drowsiness to deep sleep. REM sleep alternates with non-REM sleep at about 90 minute intervals, the first REM period lasts about 5 minutes and becomes progressively longer throughout the night, the mean length being about 15 minutes but it may last up to one hour. Rapid eye movements are only one of the characteristic features of REM sleep where muscle tone is also very much reduced, especially of the neck, chin and intercostals but sparing the diaphragm. When volunteers are deprived of REM sleep by awakening them each time they start a REM period, they make up the lost REM sleep as soon as they are permitted to do so. This may occur either later in the night or on subsequent nights when there may be prolonged REM sleep periods. In awake subjects ventilation is influenced by voluntary as well as automatic controllers, the latter being influenced by chemical (O_2 and CO_2) sensors and mechanical feedback (chest wall and airway receptors) (Cherniack, 1981). During the different sleep stages there are disturbances in the central integration of these feedback systems which cause the level of ventilation to fluctuate, notable examples being Cheyne–Stokes breathing and the sleep–apnoea syndrome. Sleep apnoea is likely when activation of the chest wall muscles exceeds that of the upper airway musculature, such as the genioglossus, so that the upper airway collapses at the beginning of inspiration. The mechanisms are outlined by Block *et al.* (1984). These effects are most likely during REM sleep when the upper airway tone is at its lowest.

The Effect of Post-operative Analgesic Regimen on Ventilatory Control

One of the problems in introducing new analgesic drugs or regimens into clinical practice is how best to evaluate their respiratory side-effects. The various conventional approaches to this problem have been reviewed recently by Drummond (1984) and McClain and Hug (1984). However, the limitations of some of these techniques when applied in the clinical environment began to become apparent during 24 hour post-operative studies in which we found that many patients who were recovering from major surgery showed periodic apnoea for several hours post-operatively (Catling *et al.*, 1980). This disturbance of ventilatory control was recognized only by continuous monitoring of breathing and was attributed to the administration of narcotic analgesics. The Respitrace inductance plethysmograph was used for the non-invasive evaluation of rib-cage and diaphragmatic movement (Tobin, 1986) but the significance of these apnoeic episodes in terms of oxygen desaturation was not realized until a later study (Catley *et al.*, 1985).

Catley *et al.* (1985) examined the interaction of sleep and analgesic regimen during a 16 hour period following major surgery under general anaesthesia.

The effects of surgery, anaesthesia and analgesic regimen on breathing patterns and oxygenation in the post-operative period were studied in two groups of patients. Each patient had received a standardized general anaesthetic and was recovering from either cholecystectomy or hip replacement. The patients were randomly allocated to receive either regional analgesia with bupivacaine or an intravenous infusion of morphine over the subsequent 24 hours and all the patients breathed air throughout the study period.

It was expected that apnoeic periods might cause a profound decrease in arterial oxygen saturation (SaO_2) when superimposed upon the common abnormality of gas exchange which persists after major surgery.

The most noticeable difference between the two groups of patients was the frequent episodes of profound oxygen desaturation in the morphine group. Patients receiving morphine had over 450 episodes of marked oxygen desaturation where SaO_2 fell below 80%; this occurred only when the ventilatory pattern was disturbed. In contrast, no patient in the post-operative regional anaesthesia group showed SaO_2 less than 87%, despite the fact that patients in this group also had apnoeic episodes (Figure 1). A surprising finding was that all the episodes of oxygen desaturation occurred only during sleep; however, REM sleep was never seen in these post-operative patients and other workers have shown that surgery may abolish REM sleep for two days post-operatively (Aurell and Elmqvist, 1985). Thus post-operative sleep apnoea is unusual in that it is induced by morphine and it occurs in the light stages of non-REM sleep. The combination of sleep, morphine and changes in circulation leads to instabilities in the ventilatory control system which manifest as sleep-related episodes of hyperventilation and apnoea independent of REM sleep. Termination of these periods of obstructive apnoea appeared to be related to partial arousal achieved at certain levels of hypoxia. If hypoxia is necessary to terminate these episodes, it would be anticipated that the administration of oxygen would prolong the apnoeic period because a longer time would be required to achieve the arousal threshold of hypoxia.

The Effects of 28% O_2 on Post-operative Ventilation and SaO_2

Both analgesic groups showed a reduced oxygen saturation post-operatively, this was more marked in the morphine group and tended to return towards normal over the subsequent 16 hours (Figure 2). In a subsequent study, a series of patients was examined during a 12 hour period following completion of surgery and anaesthesia. Oxygen was administered in the post-operative period to patients having intravenous morphine for pain relief to determine whether increasing PaO_2 either abolished the irregularity in breathing, or increased the duration but not the frequency of irregularity (Jones *et al.*, 1985).

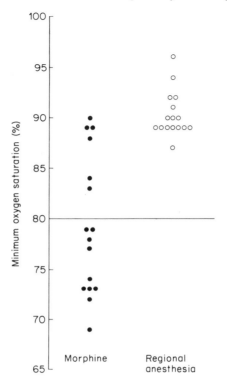

Figure 1. Shows the lowest SaO$_2$ values during sleep in the two groups of patients.

Continuous intravenous morphine was administered using the regimen described by Catley, *et al.* (1985). For successive two hour periods, patients alternately breathed air or 28% oxygen through a facemask. Using computer analysis of the ear oximeter signal, a plot was constructed of the time spent at each oxygen saturation during successive two hour periods. This clearly showed that hypoxic episodes while breathing air were abolished by the administration of oxygen. There was, however, no major effect on the number of apnoeic periods nor on the incidence of upper airway obstruction, and the duration of time spent sleeping was unaffected by the administration of oxygen. The typical effect of intermittent administration of oxygen and the time spent at a particular SaO$_2$ is shown in Figure 3 for one subject following surgery. During the 12 hour study period, there was a gradual shift to higher levels of SaO$_2$ when breathing air.

It is clear from these results that the administration of oxygen, while increasing SaO$_2$ had no beneficial effect in reducing the number of apnoeic periods.

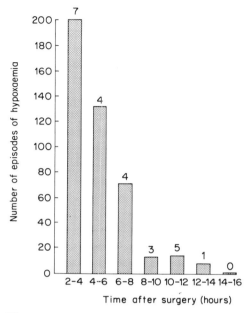

Figure 2. The number of hypoxic episodes decreases throughout the 16 hour study period.

It seems likely, therefore, that hypoxia induced by morphine is not in itself an important cause of the apnoeic periods. A more likely explanation is that it is a direct effect of morphine which during sleep causes a major disruption in ventilatory control.

Nevertheless, apnoeic episodes in the post-operative period have been seen in patients given regional anaesthesia for pain relief (Catley *et al.*, 1985) and

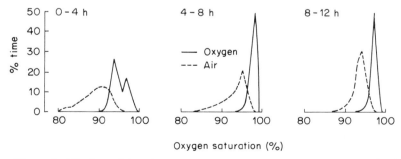

Figure 3. The beneficial effect of oxygen administration is shown. Each of the 4 hour periods was divided into two during which the patient breathed either air or 28% oxygen.

it seems likely that surgery and anaesthesia may have some lasting effects in impairing ventilatory control which gradually returns to normal. Thus the gradual diminution in the time spent at low oxygen saturation during the 12 hour study period was probably due to a waning of the effects both of the morphine loading dose and of the general anaesthetic itself. It is clear that at all times, there was a beneficial effect of oxygen administration.

Consequences of Hypoxia

Knill (personal communication) has presented evidence to support the hypothesis that the catching up period of REM sleep after surgery may occur three days later. He also showed that not only did surgery and anaesthesia abolish REM sleep for two days but the catching up night was characterized by very prolonged periods of REM sleep and profound oxygen desaturation. Jones and colleagues (1985) have postulated that these episodes of hypoxia are harmful because episodes of partial and total upper airway obstruction cause profound decreases in SaO_2 lasting up to two minutes, the lowest O_2 saturation in otherwise normal people being 72% (PaO_2 38 mmHg). Mild hypoxaemia ($SaO_2 = 85\%$ for 20 minutes) impairs short-term memory (Crow and Kelman, 1971). Patients with sleep apnoea having hypoxic episodes with a median SaO_2 of 76% showed compromised cognitive function whereas non-hypoxic sleep apnoea patients showed no such defects (Findley *et al.*, 1985). This type of repeated hypoxia may contribute to cerebral and myocardial injury in older patients with critically impaired circulation to the brain and heart. In patients with episodes of hypoxic obstructive sleep apnoea there are associated elevations of systolic blood pressure, and high values of myocardial blood flow are required to maintain the oxygen balance of the heart muscle (Shepard *et al.*, 1985). Knill (personal communication) has speculated that the third post-operative night is a particularly dangerous time and is associated with prolonged periods of hypoxia and may be the explanation for myocardial re-infarction presenting at this time in patients with a history of recent cardiac infarction within six months of surgery.

Summary

It is evident from our previous study (Catley *et al.*, 1985) that post-operative regional anaesthesia was completely free of hypoxic episodes and might prove to be the ideal form of analgesia in the patient with respiratory disease. If opiates are used, particularly with patient-demand analgesia, then it would seem wise to use a monitor either of breathing pattern or SaO_2 similar to that used in this study (Jordan, 1982). The administration of a controlled oxygen concentration appears to be beneficial. Newly available instruments for measuring beat-to-beat oxygen saturation provide an ideal monitoring device for controlling such therapy.

References

Aurell J and Elmqvist D (1985) *Br. Med. J.*, **290**, 1029–32.

Block AJ, Faulkner JA, Hughes RL, Remmers JE and Thach B (1984) *Chest*, **86**, 114–22.

Catley DM (1984) In Jones JG (ed.) Effects of Anaesthesia and Surgery on Pulmonary Mechanisms and Gas Exchange. *Int. Anesthesiol. Clin. 22*, No 4. pp 95–111, Boston: Little Brown & Co.

Catley DM, Lehane JR, Thornton C, Jordan C and Jones JG (1983) In Beneken JEW and Lavelle SM (eds) *Objective Medical Decision Making: Systems Approach to Acute Disease*. pp 209–16, Berlin: Springer-Verlag.

Catley DM, Thornton C, Jordan C, Lehane JR, Royston D and Jones JG (1985) *Anesthesiology*, **63**, 20–8.

Catling JA, Pinto DM, Jordan C and Jones JG (1980) *Br. Med. J.*, **281**, 478–80.

Cherniack NS (1981) *New Engl. J. Med.*, **305**, 325–30.

Crow TJ and Kelman GR (1971) *Br. J. Anaesth.*, **43**, 548–52.

Drummond GB (1984) In Jones JG (ed.) Effects of Anesthesia and Surgery on Pulmonary Mechanisms and Gas Exchange. *Int. Anesthesiol. Clin.* 22, No 4, 59–74. Boston: Little Brown & Co.

Findley L, Barth J, Wilholt S, Powers D, Boyd D and Surratt P (1985) *Am. Rev. Respir. Dis.*, **131**, A107.

Jones JG (1983) In Kaufman L (ed.) *Anaesthesia Review 2*, 21–38, London: Churchill Livingstone.

Jones JG, Jordan C, Scudder C, Rocke DA and Barrowcliffe M (1985) *J. R. Soc. Med.*, **78**, 1019–22.

Jordan C (1982) *Br. J. Anaesth.*, **54**, 767–82.

McClain DA and Hug DC (1984) In Jones JG (ed.) *Int. Anesthesiol. Clin. 22*, No 4, 75–94, Boston: Little Brown & Co.

Partridge MR (1984) In Kaufman L (ed.) *Anaesthesia Review 2*, 10–20, London: Churchill Livingstone.

Shepard JW, Garrison M, Grither D and Dolan GF (1985) *Am. Rev. Respir. Dis.*, **131**, A106.

Tobin MJ (1986) In Nochomovitz NL and Cherniack NS (eds) *Non-Invasive Respiratory Monitoring*. New York: Churchill Livingstone.

Aspects of Recovery from Anaesthesia
Edited by I. Hindmarch, J. G. Jones and E. Moss
© 1987 John Wiley & Sons Ltd

7

Recovery after Alfentanil Compared with Fentanyl and Volatile Agents

B. Kay

University of Manchester, Manchester

Introduction

Since its inception, general anaesthesia has usually been conducted by the use of inhalation agents, mostly vapours. Not until the introduction of methohexitone was total intravenous anaesthesia used to any great extent; the very slow elimination of thiopentone had led to instances of prolonged recovery when this agent was used to maintain anaesthesia for more than a few minutes. The introduction into clinical practice of intravenous induction agents that were eliminated more rapidly, such as methohexitone, propanidid, althesin, etomidate and propofol led to an increasing interest in using these drugs instead of volatile anaesthetics to maintain anaesthesia, particularly since concern had been voiced about pollution of the atmosphere by gaseous anaesthetics. However, use of narcotics to suppress autonomic and somatic reflex responses to surgical stimulation, mediated at spinal cord level, was always irrational and led to overdosage and underachievement; the unselective effect of the volatile anaesthetics was inevitably more effective clinically and therefore more widely used.

Since the development of the relatively short-acting opioids fentanyl, sufentanil and alfentanil, the situation has, however, changed. These drugs may be given in sufficient dosage selectively to inhibit reflex responses to surgical stimulation by reducing transmission in the nervous paths for pain transmission, specifically at the synapses in the substantia gelatinosa. Although the dose required to inhibit movement or autonomic responses is usually large, the short duration of effect of such a dose of these drugs allows their use for this purpose in many anaesthetics without leaving the patient with unacceptable post-operative respiratory depression or other unwanted effects.

The use of an opioid will usually greatly improve the quality of anaesthesia obtained from an intravenous induction agent, reducing reflex responses to surgery and at the same time, by reducing the total dose of i.v. anaesthetic, increasing the rapidity of recovery and decreasing the incidence of side-effects such as pain on injection, myoclonia, hiccough and even, paradoxically, reducing the incidence of apnoea. Thus nalbuphine and meptazinol have each been shown to improve the quality of short-term althesin and methohexitone anaesthesia (Kay *et al.*, 1984; Hargreaves *et al.*, 1985), fentanyl to reduce the total dose of thiopentone required, and shorten recovery (Epstein *et al.*, 1975), and alfentanil to improve the anaesthesia provided by althesin (Kay and Cohen, 1982).

Alfentanil improved the quality of etomidate anaesthesia (Kay and Cohen, 1983) even when N_2O, O_2 and enflurane were being given, with faster initial recovery (Colin *et al.*, 1986).

The use of alfentanil in particular with the new short-acting intravenous induction agents, has led to a much wider use of intravenous anaesthesia, and the combination has become the method of choice in some areas.

One of the main arguments put forward in favour of the new intravenous techniques has been the speed and excellent quality of recovery, and recently there has been a number of communications demonstrating this. There is, however, a dearth of comparable information regarding recovery from anaesthesia using volatile agents, where the methods have been compared concurrently, randomized and in similar circumstances. I know of no instances where double-blind assessments were made.

Pharmacokinetics and Pharmacodynamics

In the case of the intravenous induction agents and opioids there has been intensive recent research into the pharmacokinetic and pharmacodynamic aspects of the drugs mentioned.

In the majority of patients, the distribution, elimination and consequent recovery from the effects of these drugs are reasonably predictable.

Following parenteral administration, alfentanil has a low initial volume of distribution, only about 20% that of fentanyl, partly due to a lower fat solubility. This produces relatively high initial plasma concentration compared with fentanyl. In the plasma, alfentanil with a pK_a of 6.5 is 89% unionized, whereas fentanyl is only 9% unionized. The high concentration of unionized drug allows a very fast access to the receptor compartment where the receptor association/dissociation time constant for alfentanil is very short leading to a much faster onset of effect than fentanyl.

The effect is transient, due to redistribution from the plasma, with a $t_{\frac{1}{2}}\alpha$ of about 2 minutes. But the volume of distribution is again relatively small, only about 20% that of fentanyl. Alfentanil clearance is relatively low; at about

300 ml/min only half that of fentanyl, but because of the high plasma concentrations maintained due to low volumes of distribution, the amount of alfentanil eliminated is high with a $t_{\frac{1}{2}}\beta$ of about 90 minutes. It is of course broken down to inactive metabolites in the liver.

Recovery Times

There is no doubt that whatever the drugs used to maintain anaesthesia, the induction agent has a considerable effect on recovery in its immediate and subsequent aspects. Thiopentone in particular may cause a considerable delay in the recovery of normal behaviour, subjective feeling, concentration and reaction time; the work of Herbert and his colleagues (1985) showed that the effects of induction of anaesthesia by thiopentone are detectable up to the morning of the second post-operative day in contrast to the negligible effects of propofol, which has also repeatedly been shown to allow significantly faster recovery than methohexitone. In assessing the effects of opioids or volatile anaesthetics on recovery the importance of the effects of the induction agent must never be overlooked.

The use of volatile anaesthetics is characteristically associated with a slower recovery than when opiates are used to supplement anaesthesia. A standard textbook quotes recovery from the latter method as 'within two minutes' as compared with 'an average of 15 minutes' for the former (McCormack, 1980).

Not all volatile anaesthetics are the same, however, and great claims were made that the use of enflurane would allow faster recovery than when halothane was used, due to the lower blood solubility of enflurane. However, a rapid recovery after enflurane is not particularly evident in clinical use, particularly after short anaesthetics because a brief duration of exposure makes the decay curve of exhaled concentrations of an anaesthetic with high blood solubility approximate to that of an agent with lower blood solubility (Eger, 1980).

Detailed experience bears out the general opinion concerning more rapid recovery after fentanyl or alfentanil supplementation than after the use of volatile anaesthetics. Collins *et al*. (1985) compared methohexitone, N_2O and O_2 supplemented by halothane or alfentanil in 66 unpremedicated outpatients and found a mean waking time of 10.8 min (range up to 25 min) after halothane and 3.2 min after alfentanil, where the longest recovery time was 8 min. By 6 min after surgery 80% of the alfentanil group were awake and 80% of the halothane group asleep.

Antonios *et al*. (1984) showed that when alfentanil was used to supplement etomidate anaesthesia in 50 women undergoing minor gynaecological surgery the patients woke in a mean duration of 4.2 min, significantly faster than the 7.6 min required when halothane was used. The use of alfentanil also significantly reduced the incidence of the side-effects of pain on injection and myoclonia compared to the use of halothane.

Normal coin counting ability returned faster after alfentanil, and there were fewer 'p'-deletion errors 30 and 60 min post-operatively after alfentanil.

Sanders *et al*. (1984) found significantly faster recovery to opening the eyes on command and giving the correct date of birth in patients who had received alfentanil rather than halothane. Patients had a normal 'p'-deletion test 60 min post-operatively after alfentanil but not after halothane. Their 90 patients undergoing termination of pregnancy also received etomidate or methohexitone, and their results also confirmed that the use of alfentanil with etomidate provided significantly better anaesthesia with fewer side-effects than the use of halothane and etomidate.

Jellicoe (1985) demonstrated faster recovery after alfentanil than after halothane, for minor gynaecological surgery, again after induction of anaesthesia by methohexitone. Recovery to the point where the patient would give the correct date of birth and show the left thumb on request took 3.1 min after alfentanil compared to 8.4 min after halothane. The work also confirmed that the use of enflurane did not allow significantly faster recovery (8.9 min) than the use of halothane.

Cartwright (1985) compared recovery after N_2O, O_2, alfentanil or halothane in lorazepam-premedicated patients undergoing minor gynaecological or urological surgery in which anaesthesia was induced using methohexitone. Patients opened the eyes and gave their name a mean 5.6 min after alfentanil, and 10.1 min after halothane.

Short *et al*. (1985) compared alfentanil and isoflurane as supplements to methohexitone, N_2O and O_2. The patients who received alfentanil opened their eyes and gave their names and dates of birth significantly faster (4.12 min) than those who received isoflurane (9.58 min).

The use of isoflurane was also associated with a significantly higher incidence of one complication (coughing) than the use of alfentanil.

Waldron and Cookson (1984) reported the results from 643 patients observed in a multi-centre investigation. Again, patients undergoing minor surgery not involving skin incision awoke and gave their name significantly faster (3.75 min) after alfentanil supplementation of methohexitone N_2 and O_2 anaesthesia than when halothane was used (8.57 min). A similar difference (4.2 compared with 9.5 min) was noted to the time when the patient would show the left thumb on request. This study included unpremedicated patients, whilst others were premedicated with either lorazepam or temazepam. In each case, recovery was faster after alfentanil than after halothane, and in unpremedicated patients than those given premedication. The mean time to correct date of birth for unpremedicated patients receiving alfentanil was 2.6 min, compared to those who received lorazepam 5 min and

Table 1. Mean time to correct responses (min ± SEM) in patients recovering from thiopentone, N_2O and O_2 with either enflurane, fentanyl or alfentanil

Group	n	Verbal commands	Established alertness
Enflurane	19	8.1 ± 0.84	10.8 ± 0.86
Fentanyl	20	4.7 ± 0.73	7.7 ± 0.68
Alfentanil	20	2.8 ± 0.54	5.6 ± 0.52

temazepam 3.5 min. Unpremedicated patients who received halothane responded correctly after 6.4 min compared with 10 min after lorazepam and 8.5 min after temazepam.

Edelist, Haley and Aschbach (personal communication) compared enflurane with both alfentanil and fentanyl in patients undergoing short surgical procedures. The patient also received thiopentone, N_2O and O_2. They found that recovery to the time of response to verbal commands and also to the establishment of full alertness was significantly slower after enflurane than after either alfentanil or fentanyl. However, recovery to both these points was also significantly slower after fentanyl than after alfentanil (Table 1).

A number of other investigations has been carried out to compare double-blind recovery following the use of alfentanil or fentanyl in short anaesthetics. Not all these studies were able to demonstrate statistically faster recovery after alfentanil than after fentanyl, but in every instance recovery times were shorter after alfentanil. Cooper *et al.* (1983) were unable to confirm their earlier work (Sinclair and Cooper, 1983) indicating faster recovery after alfentanil than after fentanyl given at the start of methohexitone, N_2O and O_2 anaesthesia with incremental use of methohexitone; both opioids provided better anaesthesia than saline supplements.

Patrick *et al.* (1984) were also unable to demonstrate faster recovery after alfentanil than after fentanyl, again given before induction of anaesthesia by methohexitone or althesin, followed by N_2O and O_2. However, their patients who received alfentanil completed the post-box test of a later degree of recovery significantly faster (33 and 34 min) than those who received fentanyl (46 and 42 min), a finding that Cooper *et al.* (1983) did not confirm in their study. In each of these studies, groups of 20 patients were compared.

Kay and Cohen (1983) however, in a comparison of etomidate or althesin with fentanyl or alfentanil without the use of N_2O, examined groups of 40 patients and were able to demonstrate faster recovery after alfentanil than fentanyl whether measured from the last dose given (4.6 against 8.2 min) or from the end of surgery (2.1 against 5 min). The study also confirmed that alfentanil reduced the pain of etomidate injection compared with fentanyl.

Kay and Venkataraman (1983) again compared etomidate anaesthesia with either fentanyl or alfentanil in smaller groups and were unable to demonstrate statistically faster recovery after alfentanil, although the alfentanil group protruded the tongue, gave the correct name and date of birth, showed the left thumb and recovered from drowsiness in a shorter time than the fentanyl group, and also ate earlier and had less nausea and vomiting. Other tests of late recovery indicated statistically significantly faster recovery, however. Using the Maddox Wing (Hannington-Kiff, 1970), recovery of anaesthetic-induced divergence of the resting eye was significantly advanced 45 and 60 min after surgery in the alfentanil groups, with median changes of 5 and 3 dioptres respectively compared with the fentanyl group, median changes of 8 and 7 dioptres. Using Wechsler's digit substitution test (Wechsler, 1944), performance was diminished for only 30 min after alfentanil, but for 60 min after fentanyl, and there was a significant difference between the groups at each time. The results confirm results (Patrick *et al.*, 1984) indicating a faster return to normal at later stages of recovery after alfentanil compared with fentanyl.

Kallar and Keenan (1984) also found a significantly shorter median time (13 min) to 'complete recovery' after alfentanil than after fentanyl (35 min).

On the other hand, Kennedy and Ogg (1985) were unable to demonstrate any difference in recovery and memory function between fentanyl and alfentanil. However, they gave the opioid two minutes before induction of anaesthesia, and subsequently gave increments of methohexitone, which is not the best drug for controlling reflex responses to anaesthesia, as we have noted.

To obtain the best results using alfentanil for minor surgery of short duration, the drug must be given in small doses, e.g. 4 μg/kg^{-1} initially and 2 μg/kg^{-1} subsequently, slowly enough to prevent the occurrence of apnoea, i.e. over about 15 sec, but frequently enough, approximately each minute, to build up and maintain an effect appropriate to the clinical situation. It must be remembered that the effect will be apparent about a minute after i.v. injection and will continue for a further 3–4 min. Administration may usually be ended several minutes before the end of surgery, hastening recovery and reducing side-effects. Benzodiazepines, which add to respiratory depression and delay recovery should be avoided, and the intravenous induction agent given in the minimum amounts that will induce and maintain unawareness, remembering the hypnotic effect of the alfentanil. N_2O should be avoided; our own experience agrees with that of Alexander *et al.* (1984) and Lonie and Harper (1986) N_2O causes post-operative nausea and vomiting. Propofol is the best i.v. anaesthetic for these short anaesthetics, allowing faster recovery than any other, with waking as fast as after N_2O. The combination of propofol and alfentanil can provide excellent anaesthesia with fast recovery, few side-effects and total patient satisfaction (Kay *et al.*, 1986). It is my method of choice for all minor surgery of short duration.

References

Alexander GD, Skupski JN and Brown EM (1984) The role of N_2O in post-operative nausea and vomiting. *Anesth. Analg.*, **63**, 175.

Antonios WRA, Inglis MD and Lees NW (1984) Alfentanil in minor gynaecological surgery: use with etomidate and a comparison with halothane. *Anaesthesia*, **39**, 812–5.

Cartwright DP (1985) Recovery after anaesthesia with alfentanil or halothane. *Can. Anaesth. Soc. J.*, **32**, 479–83.

Colin RIW, Drummond GB and Spence AA (1986) Alfentanil supplemented anaesthesia for short procedures. *Anaesthesia*, **41**, 477–81.

Collins KM, Plantevin OM, Whitburn RH and Doyle JP (1985) Outpatient termination of pregnancy: halothane or alfentanil-supplemented anaesthesia. *Br. J. Anaesth.*, **57**, 1226–31.

Cooper GM, O'Conner M, Mark J and Harvey J (1983) Effect of alfentanil and fentanyl on recovery from brief anaesthesia. *Br. J. Anaesth.*, **55**, 179S.

Eger EI (1980) Inhalation anaesthesia: pharmacokinetics. In Gray TC, Nunn JF and Utting JE (eds) *General Anaesthesia I*, 4th Edn. p. 90. London: Butterworths.

Epstein B, Levy ML, Thein M and Cookley C (1975) Evaluation of fentanyl as an adjunct to thiopentone N_2O–O_2 anaesthesia for short surgical procedures. *Anesthesiol. Rev.*, **2**, 24–9.

Hannington-Kiff JG (1970) Measurement of recovery from outpatient general anaesthesia with a simple ocular test. *Br. Med. J.*, **3**, 132–5.

Hargreaves J, Kay B and Healy TEJ (1985) Meptazinol as an analgesic adjunct to total intravenous anaesthesia in cystoscopy patients. *Anaesthesia*, **40**, 490–3.

Herbert M, Matain SW, Bourne JB and Hart EA (1985) Recovery of mental abilities following general anaesthesia induced by propofol or thiopentone. *Postgrad. Med. J.*, **61**, 53, 132.

Jellicoe JA (1985) A comparison of alfentanil, halothane and enflurane for day case gynaecological surgery. *Anaesthesia*, **40**, 810–2.

Kallar SK and Keenan RL (1984) Evaluation and comparison of recovery time from alfentanil and fentanyl for short surgical procedures. *Anesthesiology*, **61**, A379.

Kay B and Cohen AT (1982) Althesin and alfentanil for minor surgery. In Prys-Roberts C, Vickers MD (eds) *Cardiovascular Measurement in Anaesthesiology*. p 104. Berlin: Springer-Verlag.

Kay B and Cohen AT (1983) Intravenous anaesthesia for minor surgery. *Br. J. Anaesth.*, **55**, 165S–7S.

Kay B, Hargreaves J and Healy TEJ (1984) Nalbuphine and Althesin anaesthesia. *Anaesthesia*, **39**, 666–9.

Kay B, Hargreaves J, Sivalingam T and Healy TEJ (1986) Intravenous anaesthesia for cystoscopy. *Eur. J. Anaesthesiol.*, **3**, 111–20.

Kay B and Venkataraman P (1983) Recovery after fentanyl and alfentanil in anaesthesia for minor surgery. *Br. J. Anaesth.*, **55**, 169S–71S.

Kennedy DJ and Ogg TW (1985) Alfentanil and memory function. *Anaesthesia*, **40**, 537–40.

Lonie DS and Harper NJN (1986) Nitrous oxide anaesthesia and vomiting. *Anaesthesia*, **41**, 703–8.

McCormack RS (1980) Post-operative recovery. In Gray TC, Nunn JF and Utting JE, (eds) *General Anaesthesia II* 4th Ed. p. 1065. London: Butterworths.

Patrick M, Egar BM, Toft DF and Sebel PS (1984) Alfentanil supplemented anaesthesia for short procedures. *Br. J. Anaesth.*, **56**, 861–5.

Sanders RS, Sinclair ME and Sear JW (1984) Alfentanil in short procedures. *Anaesthesia*, **39**, 1202–6.

Short SM, Rutherford CF and Sebel PS (1985) A comparison between isoflurane and alfentanil supplemented anaesthesia for short procedures. *Anaesthesia*, **40**, 1160–4.

Sinclair M and Cooper GM (1983) Alfentanil and recovery. *Anaesthesia*, **38**, 435.

Waldron HA and Cookson RF (1984) Use of a viewdata system to collect data from a multi-centre clinical trial in anaesthesia. *Br. Med. J.*, **289**, 1059–61.

Wechsler D (1944) *The Measurement of Adult Intelligence* p. 185. Baltimore: Williams & Wilkins.

Aspects of Recovery from Anaesthesia
Edited by I. Hindmarch, J. G. Jones and E. Moss

8

A Comparison of Recovery after Halothane or Alfentanil in Anaesthesia for Minor Surgery

E. Moss[1], *I. Hindmarch*[2], *A. J. Pain*[2], *R. S. Edmonson*[1]

[1]*The General Infirmary, Leeds* [2]*The University of Leeds, Leeds*

(This is an abstract of a paper published in the *British Journal of Anaesthesia* **59**, 970–977 (1987) and is printed with the permission of the Editor.)

Introduction

One of the requirements for an ideal technique of anaesthesia for day case surgery is the rapid attainment of street fitness. The synthetic opioid, alfentanil, has a rapid onset and short duration of action (Niegmegeers and Janssen, 1981; Sinclair and Cooper, 1983) and has great potential for use in day stay patients. The results of published work on rate of recovery following alfentanil have been conflicting, so this investigation was carried out to compare the rate of recovery following an anaesthetic technique which employed alfentanil with that after a popular anaesthetic combination (intravenous methohexitone, nitrous oxide and halothane). Methohexitone was used because this was the only suitable intravenous anaesthetic agent available at the time of the study. The physical and mental aspects of recovery were studied over a 19 hour period following anaesthesia.

Methods

Ethical Committee approval for the study was obtained and 44 patients (ASA grades I and II) undergoing dilatation and curettage and/or cystoscopy gave their informed consent. No pre-operative medication was given and the patients were randomly allocated to two groups. In the halothane group, anaesthesia was induced with methohexitone and maintained with nitrous oxide, oxygen and halothane 1–1.5%. The alfentanil group received alfentanil 0.25 mg then anaesthesia was induced with methohexitone and maintained with nitrous oxide (66%), oxygen (33%) and alfentanil 0.25 mg one minute before surgery commenced and at five minute intervals thereafter to a maximum dose of 1 mg. Increments of methohexitone were given as required.

Familiarization with the test procedures and recording of baseline scores took place 3–4 hours before surgery which occurred between 14.00 and 15.00 h. Testing took place in a room off the main ward to standardize lighting and noise levels. Post-operative tests were performed at 45, 75, 120 and 180 min after discontinuation of the anaesthetic gases, and again at 19 h. Any period of intra-operative apnoea lasting more than 20 sec was noted and paracetamol 1 g was given for post-operative analgesia if required. The test procedures included:

The Maddox Wing (MW) which measures the balance of extraocular muscle activity. The fusion mechanism of the eyes is impaired by centrally acting drugs and deviation of the eyes is accentuated.

The critical flicker fusion test (CFF) which measures the ability to distinguish discrete sensory information and is an index of cortical activity. The mean threshold of the flicker fusion was the score used at each test for three ascending trials, where the discrete flashes of light become continuous, and three descending trials, where the apparently continuous light becomes discrete flashes.

The choice reaction time (CRT) is a measure of sensori-motor performance (Hindmarch and Subhan, 1983) in which three types of reaction time are automatically recorded. These are the recognition reaction time (RRT), the time taken to lift the index finger from a rest template in response to a light stimulus, the total reaction time (TRT), the time taken to reach the appropriate response button, and the motor response time (MRT) which is the difference between these two times.

Line analogue rating scales (LARS) (Hindmarch and Gudgeon, 1980) were used to measure perceived sedation.

The tracking test measures patients' ability to use a joystick to track a moving arrow on a television screen. The mean distance between the tips of the target and tracking arrows over a one minute period was the measure used. A 'peripheral awareness' task was also included in which the subject was asked to react to a stimulus presented in the periphery of vision (Hindmarch, Subhan and Stoker, 1983).

A semantic memory test in which the patient was required to categorize test words so that information processing could be studied.

The last two computer based tests were not used until the 2 hour test.

Results

From 44 patients who consented to participate in the trial, 40 completed all the post-operative testing. The two anaesthetic groups were comparable with regard to age and weight of the patients and the duration of anaesthesia. When comparing the two groups, immediate recovery was found to be faster in the alfentanil group ($P < 0.01$), but apnoea ($P < 0.05$) and hiccoughs ($P < 0.05$) were more common than in the halothane group. The CFF test showed that on the morning following, the alfentanil patients were less sedated ($P < 0.05$), but all the other tests showed no difference between the groups. The CFF test proved to be the most sensitive test of recovery as it remained significantly depressed in both groups at 3 h after anaesthesia. In contrast, the MW and CRT scores were significantly depressed at 2 h, but had returned to normal by 3 h. In the tracking test and semantic memory test, there appeared to be a practice effect; scores were significantly depressed at 2 h and returned to normal by 3 h. The LARS scores showed an initial increase in sedation scores which gradually reduced until the following morning when they were slightly less than normal. There was no difference in perceived sedation between the groups.

Summary

The findings of this investigation broadly agree with those of other workers (for references see Moss *et al.*, 1987) in that immediate recovery was more rapid with alfentanil but later recovery was similar to that with other anaesthetic techniques. Intra-operative apnoea occurred more frequently with alfentanil than with halothane but provided the airway is carefully assessed before anaesthesia, this can be treated easily by manual ventilation via a mask. Episodic apnoea was less of a problem as the study progressed suggesting that the problem is reduced when the anaesthetist is more familiar with the technique. Some tests of recovery were still impaired at 3 h after the end of anaesthesia, which confirms the need to warn patients not to perform any tasks requiring unimpaired concentration for at least 24 h following anaesthesia to allow a margin of safety.

The tests of recovery used in this study have been shown to reflect impairment of psychomotor function reliably (Hindmarch and Bhatti, this volume). The CFF test is particularly sensitive to impairment of higher intellectual function.

From this study, we can conclude that immediate recovery is faster with alfentanil but there is essentially no difference between the groups in later tests, apnoea is more common with alfentanil, the CFF test is, in this situation, the best measure of post-anaesthetic recovery, and an anaesthetic technique using methohexitone and alfentanil is suitable for day case anaesthesia.

Since this study was completed, a new intravenous anaesthetic, propofol, has been released. In the author's hands, this has proved easier to use in combination with alfentanil than methohexitone, providing better operating conditions and rapid awakening.

References

Hindmarch I and Gudgeon AC (1980) The effects of clobazam and lorazepam on aspects of psychomotor performance and car handling ability. *Br. J. Clin. Pharmacol.*, **10**, 145–50.

Hindmarch I and Subhan Z (1983) The effects of midazolam in conjunction with alcohol on sleep, psychomotor performance and car driving ability. *Int. J. Clin. Pharmacol. Res. III*, **5**, 323–9.

Hindmarch I, Subhan Z and Stoker M (1983) The effects of amitriptyline on car driving and psychomotor performance. *Acta Psychiatr. Scand.* Suppl 308, **68**, 141–6.

Moss E, Hindmarch I, Pain AJ and Edmonson RS (1987) A comparison of recovery after halothane or alfentanil in anaesthesia for minor surgery. *Br. J. Anaesth.*, **59**, 970–7.

Niegmegeers CJE and Janssen PAJ (1981) Alfentanil (R 392090): A particularly short-acting intravenous narcotic analgesic in rats. *Drug Development Research*, **1**, 83–8.

Sinclair ME and Cooper GM (1983) Alfentanil and recovery. *Anaesthesia*, **38**, 435–7.

Aspects of Recovery from Anaesthesia
Edited by I. Hindmarch, J. G. Jones and E. Moss
© 1987 John Wiley & Sons Ltd

9

Recovery after Propofol

T. E. J. Healy

University of Manchester, Manchester

In his memorable classic *On the Inhalation of the Vapour of Ether* which was published in 1847, John Snow described many of the salient features of general anaesthesia that we recognize and accept today. He noted that 'Elderly people are slower in recovering than young ones' and 'Although many patients recover their consciousness at once, as out of a natural sleep, yet there is often a short period during which the mind wanders'. He also drew attention to the occurrence of vomiting, nausea and respiratory depression in the initial post-operative period. Thus an interest in a rapid and uncomplicated recovery is not new, but has been of concern to anaesthetists from the very beginnings of our speciality. Indeed, many patients still express a particular anxiety about the possibility of not recovering from anaesthesia.

There are a number of different techniques now available for inducing general anaesthesia. The latest drug to be made available is propofol, which, because of its low solubility in water, was prepared in Cremophor EL. However, adverse reactions to cremophor occurred and it has now been made available in an aqueous emulsion in soya bean oil and purified egg phosphatide. Propofol has several useful properties such as a rapid and smooth onset of effect, short duration, minimal accumulation, rapid clear-headed recovery and few excitatory effects. It does not alter ganglionic transmission.

Whereas histamine release occurred following injection of the cremophor preparation, it does not occur following injection of the emulsion preparation. Most of the propofol metabolites are excreted in the urine. Cumulation of propofol is probably very minimal when compared with cumulation of thiopentone. Pharmacokinetic studies show that plasma propofol concentration following a bolus injection declines exponentially and can be described using a three compartment model. The half-life for the first phase is approximately three minutes which is consistent with redistribution of the drug. The second phase has a half-life of approximately 45 minutes and is due to metabolism. The initial volume of distribution is much greater than the actual body volume and is, of course, an aqueous equivalent volume. The systemic whole blood clearance is much greater than the liver blood flow suggesting a metabolic pathway in addition to that in the liver. Indeed, the lack of cumulation with multiple doses together with rapid clearance is consistent with subsequent rapid awakening.

No important differences in the derived kinetic indices for male and female patients have been shown (Kay *et al*., 1986a) and the presence of renal failure does not influence clearance. An interesting notch occurs in the whole blood–time concentration curve at the time of awakening (Kay *et al*., 1986b). This is thought to be due to a change in circulation to poorly perfused regions, which occurs at this time.

The speed of induction of anaesthesia is not altered by the administration of benzodiazepine operatively. The duration of anaesthesia resulting from a bolus injection of propofol has been examined (Nightingale *et al*., 1985). Loss of consciousness occurred within a mean of 26 seconds, episodic apnoea and a relative hypotension being the most notable side-effects.

The frontalis EMG was used to indicate sleep and recovery. The change in the pattern of the frontalis EMG has been shown to be an excellent indicator of emergence from induction (Kay *et al*., 1982). The mean duration of unconsciousness measured from the start of injection to reappearance of EMG activity was 7.4 minutes. We could, therefore, expect that propofol might have a sufficiently short duration of action to make it suitable for outpatient use.

Sixty patients who were to undergo cystoscopy as outpatients have been studied (Kay *et al*., 1986a). Patients were given either methohexitone 1.5 mg/kg or propofol 2 mg/kg following alfentanil 7 μg/kg. Anaesthesia was then maintained using the same drugs used to induce anaesthesia. The patients in each of the groups were well matched while the induction doses of the two drugs were similar as were the duration of anaesthesia and the total doses of methohexitone and propofol required to maintain anaesthesia. However, the pattern of recovery after propofol is more rapid than after methohexitone when assessed using simple tests, e.g. times to eyes open or tongue protruded on command. These results were confirmed using a digit substitution test and eye divergence using the Maddox Wing.

In another study, Mackenzie and Grant (1985) compared recovery after thiopentone 5 mg/kg, methohexitone 1.5 mg/kg and propofol 2.5 mg/kg. Anaesthesia was maintained with nitrous oxide and enflurane. The duration of surgery was similar in the three groups in their study. The recovery assessments, i.e. time to open eyes and repeat date of birth suggested a more rapid recovery after propofol.

The more sensitive psychometric tests, i.e. choice reaction time and critical flicker fusion, suggested a significantly more rapid recovery after propofol.

Patients who received propofol showed no impairment at 30 minutes after anaesthesia apart from the motor component of the choice reaction time. However, patients who received thiopentone showed a significantly slower recovery and performance was still impaired at the 90 minute test.

Further evidence for the rapid recovery after propofol has been given by Herbert *et al.* (1985).

Day case surgery requiring anaesthesia is likely to increase in popularity. In this context, an anaesthetic agent which allows a rapid recovery of street fitness will prove very useful.

References

Herbert M, Makin SW, Bourke JB and Hart EA (1985) Recovery of mental abilities following general anaesthesia induced by propofol (Diprivan) or thiopentone. *Postgrad. Med. J.*, **61**, Suppl 3, 132.

Kay B, Hargreaves J and Healy TEJ (1982) Combined electro-encephalography (EEG) and electromyography (EMG) for measurement of depth of anaesthesia. In *Proceedings of the European Academy of Anaesthesiology*, pp 136–141. Berlin: Springer-Verlag.

Kay B, Hargreaves J, Sivalingam T and Healy TEJ (1986a) Intravenous anaesthesia for cystoscopy: a comparison of propofol or methohexitone with alfentanil. *Eur. J. Anaesthesiol.*, **3**, 111–20.

Kay NH, Sear JW, Uppington J, Cockshott ID and Douglas EJ (1986b) Disposition of propofol in patients undergoing surgery. A comparison of men and women. *Br. J. Anaesth.*, **58**, 1075–9.

Mackenzie N and Grant IS (1985) Comparison of the new emulsion formulation of propofol with methohexitone and thiopentone for induction of anaesthesia in day cases. *Br. J. Anaesth.*, **57**, 725–31.

Nightingale P, Healy TEJ, Hargreaves J, McGuinness K and Kay B (1985) Propofol in emulsion form: induction characteristics and venous sequelae. *Eur. J. Anaesthesiol.* **2**, 361–8.

Aspects of Recovery from Anaesthesia
Edited by I. Hindmarch, J. G. Jones and E. Moss
© 1987 John Wiley & Sons Ltd

10

The Effects of Benzodiazepines on Recovery

J. W. Dundee

The Queen's University of Belfast, Belfast

Introduction

There are no reliable controlled studies comparing recovery times from benzodiazepines and other anaesthetic agents. It is a clinical impression that the action of benzodiazepine seems more prolonged than that of thiopentone, methohexitone or the more recently introduced propofol but there are no data to quantify this difference.

Before looking in detail at recovery from benzodiazepines, it is helpful to consider their uses in anaesthetic practice. The benzodiazepines most commonly used by anaesthetists are listed in Table 1. Some of the clinical indications are shown in Table 2. Most anaesthetists would agree that there is a role for the benzodiazepines in pre-anaesthetic medication although there will be differences as to the choice of drug. For night-time hypnotics, particularly on the night before operation, many would use long-acting drugs such as lorazepam or nitrazepam but some would prefer the shorter acting drug, temazepam. It is their role in the induction of anaesthesia which probably causes most controversy particularly comparing practice in Britain with continental Europe and North America. Some North American workers (Reves *et al.*, 1979) recommend the soluble benzodiazepines as induction agents and likewise there is a vogue for their use for this purpose in continental Europe, where flunitrazepam is very popular.

However, the author and colleagues have not found the benzodiazepines to be as reliable as the barbiturates for induction of anaesthesia and would only recommend their use in elderly patients (Dundee *et al.*, 1986b), in conjunction with opioid premedication or following immediate pretreatment with opioids: even in these circumstances midazolam was not proved fully reliable in young patients (Dundee *et al.*, 1986c). The use of benzodiazepines for

61

Table 1. Benzodiazepines most commonly used
by anaesthetists

Oral	Injectable
Diazepam	Diazepam—Valium
Flunitrazepam†	—Diazemuls
Lorazepam*	Flunitrazepam†
Midazolam	Midazolam
Nitrazepam	(Lorazepam*)
Oxazepam	
Clobazam	

* Although lorazepam is available in injectable form
this is not used for induction of anaesthesia, but may
be used as a sedative-hypnotic.
† Not available in injectable form in Britain.

maintenance of anaesthesia is in an experimental stage and can be largely
ignored.

It is in the field of sedation that the injectable benzodiazepines have their
main use. Many patients who would not accept local anaesthesia will be
prepared to do so after sedation with a small dose of diazepam or midazolam
and this applies particularly in the field of endoscopy or dental procedures. It
may be that here the effect of the benzodiazepines on memory are put to their
best use because of the intense amnesic action shortly after intravenous
injection, so that the patient does not recall the injection of a local anaesthetic
or the passing of an endoscope. Their use in intensive care is widely accepted
and recently there have been studies on their use as infusions both in the
intensive care unit and in the post-operative period after cardiac operations.
The anticonvulsant action of these drugs has been included in Table 2 for the
sake of completeness and there are some data to suggest that they might have

Table 2. Uses of benzodiazepines in anaesthetic
practice

> Preanaesthetic medication
> Night time hypnotic
> Induction of anaesthesia
> (Maintenance of anaesthesia)
> Sedation—with local anaesthesia
>   —in the intensive care unit
>   —postoperative
> Anticonvulsant
> (Antiemetic)

an antiemetic action but these are not important indications. It is when used as pre-anaesthetic medication, as night-time hypnotic or for induction of anaesthesia, that one is concerned with the effect of the benzodiazepines on recovery.

Metabolism and Recovery

By looking at the pharmacokinetics and metabolism of the different groups of drugs one can draw conclusions which are helpful in assessing the effect of benzodiazepines on recovery.

The rapidity of recovery from intravenous thiopentone or methohexitone is mainly attributable to rapid translocation in the body and consequent removal from the nervous system. It is only after repeat administration or the use of very large doses, that detoxication plays a major part in early recovery.

Hudson, Stanski and Burch (1982) have shown that the elimination half-life of thiopentone is about 11 h compared with 4 h for methohexitone. These times are both longer than for midazolam (2–5 h), yet there is a much more rapid early recovery from either barbiturate compared with the benzodiazepine. This must be due to the very rapid early distribution with t'B in the region of 6–8 min for both barbiturates which is much shorter than that of any of the benzodiazepines (Collier *et al.*, 1982).

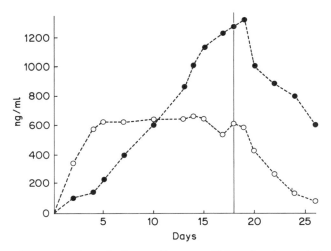

Figure 1. Typical plasma diazepam (○) and n-desmethyl diazepam (●) levels following 10 mg iv 4 hourly over a prolonged period. Continuous line shows when drug therapy discontinued. (Reproduced by courtesy of *British Journal of Anaesthesia*)

The major route for the metabolism of thiopentone is to a carboxylic acid derivative which is inactive. This is in sharp contrast with the metabolism of diazepam to the n-desmethyl derivative which has a prolonged hypnotic effect. Hydroxylation is an alternative but less important route for diazepam and is the only mechanism available for the neonate. After repeated administration, there is accumulation of the hypnotically active metabolite of diazepam because it has a much slower elimination rate than the parent compound.

An example of this is shown in Figure 1, which shows the plasma concentration of both diazepam and n-desmethyl diazepam in a patient who was given 10 mg diazepam 4-hourly for 17 days (Gamble *et al.*, 1976). Return of consciousness after stopping diazepam took 4–5 days in this patient. In this patient, the elimination of half-life was about 6 days for diazepam and 10–12 days for the metabolite, suggesting some saturation of the detoxication process after large doses. By now physicians should know of the cumulative effect of repeated doses of diazepam and avoid delay in recovery by reducing both the frequency of administration and the dose of drug used.

Table 3 shows some of the differences between diazepam and midazolam which are important in relation to recovery. Note the lack of a hypnotically active metabolite with midazolam (Dundee *et al.*, 1984). More important is the shorter elimination half-life of midazolam. With both drugs there is a relationship between age of the patient and elimination half-life which is prolonged in the elderly. This is not important with single clinical doses, nor does it necessarily indicate an increased sensitivity to the drug in the elderly. It could be important on repeat administration where recovery in the elderly may be prolonged.

It is of some interest to note that hypnotically active metabolites are

Table 3. Physical and pharmocokinetic differences between diazepam and midazolam

	Diazepam	Midazolam
Water solubility	–	+
Relative potency	1	1.6–2.0
Protein binding	97–98%	95–96%
Lipophilicity	×5–10	1
Hypnotically active metabolite	Yes	No
Elimination half-life (h)		
Young	15–20	2–3
Elderly	20–50	4–8
Second peak effect	obvious	minimal

(from Dundee *et al.*, 1984).

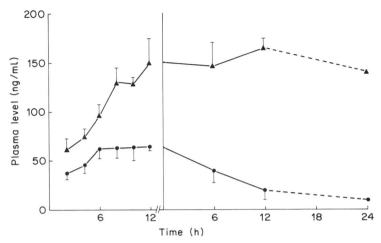

Figure 2. Trough plasma diazepam (▲) and midazolam (●) levels (ng/ml⁻¹) associated with 2-hourly administration of 5 mg doses given to patients following open heart surgery and declining levels following discontinuation of medication (Lowry *et al.*, 1985). (Reproduced by courtesy of *British Journal of Anaesthesia*)

produced following the administration of medazepam, chlordiazepoxide, demoxapam, prazepam, chlorazepate and flurazepam. In contrast, temazepam, oxazepam and clobazam are end-products with no hypnotically active metabolites. Recovery following the latter will be more complete than after drugs with an active metabolite because the parent drug is eliminated.

Figure 2 compares plasma levels of diazepam and midazolam when these are given at 2-hourly intervals following open heart surgery. With diazepam, there is a greater rise in plasma concentration while recovery after midazolam is much shorter than after diazepam.

This rapidity of recovery has been noted when patients after cardiac operations were given an infusion of midazolam 2 mg per hour (Dundee *et al.*, 1986d). This produced very good sedation and constant plasma level in the region of 80–100 ng/ml⁻¹. When the infusion was discontinued, the elimination half-life of the drug was not much longer than that following a single-dose in young patients, averaging between 5 and 6 h. Recovery occurred within one hour which is much better than after diazepam.

In our cardiac surgery study, we found one patient in whom the plasma midazolam concentration continued to rise for 8–10 h indicating atypically slow metabolism. In this patient, clearance was only 236 ml/kg/h compared with an average of 350 in the remaining patients in this study. In a study of pharmacokinetics in over 200 patients given a standard dose of 0.3 mg/kg⁻¹

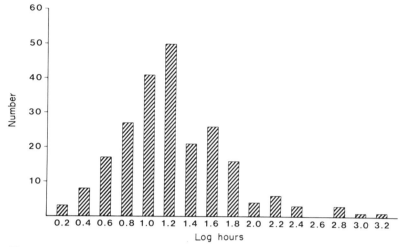

Figure 3. Scatter of elimination half lives in over 200 adults given 0.3 mg/kg^{-1} midazolam iv (calculated from Dundee *et al.*, 1986a).

midazolam, 1 : 20 had an abnormal elimination half-life as shown in Figure 3 (Dundee *et al.*, 1986d). This is not of clinical importance for single doses but is very important when one looks at recovery from repeated administrations or infusions. Perhaps this will explain some of the delayed recovery cases reported in correspondence in various medical journals. While this has been demonstrated with midazolam, it may occur with all the benzodiazepines.

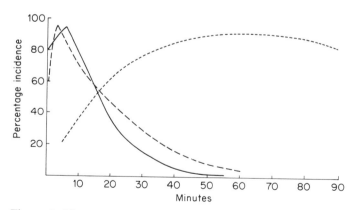

Figure 4. The extent and duration of amnesia following equipotent intravenous doses of 5 mg midazolam (——), 10 mg diazepam (– –) and 4 mg lorazepam (- - -) (from Dundee and Pandit, 1972; Dundee and Wilson, 1980; George and Dundee, 1976).

One final point relating to recovery is the possibility of amnesia persisting into the post-operative period. A short period of anterograde amnesia follows single intravenous doses of diazepam, flunitrazepam and midazolam, in contrast with the very prolonged amnesia following equivalent doses of lorazepam (Figure 4). The importance of the letter is obvious when giving advice to patients in the immediate post-operative period.

References

Collier PS, Kawar P, Gamble JAS and Dundee JW (1982) Influence of age on pharmacokinetics of midazolam. *Br. J. Clin. Pharmacol.*, **13**, 602P.

Dundee JW, Collier PS, Carlisle RJT and Harper KW (1986a) Prolonged midazolam elimination half-life. *Br. J. Clin. Pharmacol.*, **21**, 425–30.

Dundee JW and George KA (1976) The amnesic action of diazepam, flunitrazepam and lorazepam in man. *Acta Anaesthesiol. Belg.* **27**, suppl. 3–11.

Dundee JW, Halliday NJ and Harper KW (1986b) Midazolam as an intravenous induction agent in the elderly. *Anesth. Analg.*, **65**, 1089–90.

Dundee JW, Halliday NJ, Harper KW and Brogden RN (1984) Midazolam: a review of its pharmacological properties and therapeutic use. *Drugs*, **28**, 519–43.

Dundee JW, Halliday NJ, McMurray TJ and Harper KW (1986c) Pretreatment with opioids. The effect on thiopentone induction requirements and on the onset of action of midazolam. *Anaesthesia*, **41**, 159–61.

Dundee JW, Mathews HML, Carson IW, Orr IA, Lyons SM and Clarke RSJ (1986d) Midazolam sedation following open heart surgery. In Bergmann H, Kramar H, Steinbereithner (eds) *Beitrage zue Anaesthesiologie und Intensivmedizin 17*. Abstracts II or VII European Congress of Anaesthesiology, Vienna, 7–13 September 1986, p 18. Maudrich, Vienna.

Dundee JW and Pandit SK (1972) Studies on drug induced amnesia with intravenous anaesthetic agents in man. *Br. J. Clin. Pract.* **26**, 164–9.

Dundee JW and Wilson DB (1980) Amnesic action of midazolam. *Anaesthesia*, **35**, 459–61.

Gamble JAS, Dundee JW and Gray RC (1976) Plasma diazepam concentrations following prolonged administration. *Br. J. Anaesth.*, **48**, 1087–90.

Hudson RJ, Stanski DR and Burch PA (1982) Comparative pharmacokinetics of methohexital and thiopental. *Anesthesiology*, **57**, A420.

Lowry KG, Dundee JW, McClean E, Lyons SM, Carson IW and Orr IA (1985) Pharmacokinetics of diazepam and midazolam when used for sedation following cardiopulmonary bypass. *Br. J. Anaesth.*, **57**, 883–5.

Reves JC, Vinik R, Hirschfield AM, Holcomb C and Strong S (1979) Midazolam compared with thiopentone as a hypnotic component in balanced anaesthesia. A randomised, double-blind study. *Can. Anaesth. Soc. J.*, **26**, 42–9.

Aspects of Recovery from Anaesthesia
Edited by I. Hindmarch, J. G. Jones and E. Moss
© 1987 John Wiley & Sons Ltd

11

After-effects of Benzodiazepines in Gynaecological Surgery

C. G. Male

University of Keele, Stoke-on-Trent

Introduction

The attractions of benzodiazepine drugs for pre-operative medication include relief of anxiety, amnesia, sedation, anticonvulsant properties and the absence of respiratory depression. The oral route which is preferred by patients, leads to a sustained peak effect which permits a variable time between medication and operation. Disadvantages of benzodiazepines in this context would include prolonged duration and variability of effect, lack of antiemetic effect, and possible anti-analgesic properties.

Methods

All observations and comments on the after-effects of benzodiazepines are based on two studies of in-patients undergoing minor gynaecological surgery in Christchurch, New Zealand (Male *et al.*, 1980) and Stoke-on-Trent, UK (Male and Johnson, 1984).

The protocols shared many features; common entry criteria for the patients included being an adult female caucasian, within a limited range of body weight, with a haemoglobin concentration above 10 g/dl, ASA grade I or II, free from pain requiring potent analgesic therapy and about to undergo minor gynaecological surgery.

A standard anaesthetic technique with intravenous thiopentone induction and maintenance with nitrous oxide, oxygen, and halothane was employed for the short procedure.

The average age in the first study was 31 years, compared with 41 years in the second. Weight, height, anaesthetic fitness and pre-operative haemoglobin concentrations were comparable.

The first study was designed to identify the relative potency of oral flunitrazepam and to compare its suitability for premedication with diazepam and lorazepam. The second study investigated the early recovery from oxazepam and clobazam when compared with diazepam and lorazepam under similar circumstances. Both studies were randomized, double-blind, and placebo controlled. Assessments were made before and one hour after oral premedication and within 16 to 24 hours after operation. Additional assessments were made two and four hours after operation in the UK study. The observer gave scores for drowsiness and apprehension on a scale 0 to 3 and excitement on a scale 0 to 2 after Dundee *et al.* (1962). Dizziness, emesis and headache were graded by questioning the patient.

To identify that group of patients particularly in need of anxiolysis, we used the self-rating multiple effect adjective check-list of Zuckerman (1960) reduced to 11 anxiety-present and 10 anxiety-absent words. These were displayed on cards in large print and the patient was asked to choose those words which best described her feelings at that moment. An Eysenck personality inventory was completed by the patient before premedication and after operation to evaluate aspects of personality that might influence the success of the drug therapy. Thirty patients were assigned to each drug group, but in New Zealand, we compared moderate and high doses of diazepam, lorazepam and flunitrazepam, whereas in the UK, we chose single moderate doses of diazepam, lorazepam, oxazepam and clobazam.

Results

In the first study, observer rating of drowsiness, one hour after premedication, showed significant ($P < 0.01$) drug effect with flunitrazepam 1 mg and lorazepam 2.5 mg inducing greater drowsiness than the placebo but doubling the dose failed to increase the drowsiness significantly. Drowsiness 16–24 hours after premedication showed a significant difference ($P < 0.01$) across the groups principally due to the moderate and high doses of lorazepam.

In the second project, observer rating of drowsiness showed that 60 min after premedication, there was a significant increase in drowsiness ($P < 0.01$) with diazepam 10 mg having a greater effect than clobazam 10 mg, oxazepam 30 mg or placebo. These differences were not found using patient self-rating scores for drowsiness. However, there were significant correlations between observer and self-rating scores for drowsiness ($r = 0.86$ and 0.75), excitement/relaxation ($r = 0.77$ and 0.81), and anxiety ($r = 0.73$ and 0.59). Two and four hours after operation, lorazepam 2 mg produced significantly ($P < 0.01$) more drowsiness than the other four groups. No differences were apparent the day after operation.

For the observer rating of apprehension in New Zealand patients, only flunitrazepam 1 mg achieved significant relief of apprehension compared with placebo ($P < 0.01$). Doubling the doses of the other benzodiazepines failed to relieve apprehension further. The correlation coefficients between observer and self-rating scores for anxiety were $r = 0.51$ before and $r = 0.30$ after premedication. Although highly significantly different from zero, the coefficients are not very great.

For the observer rating of apprehension in UK patients, no significant differences were manifest between the drug groups. Though showing more apprehension than their New Zealand counterparts before premedication, this was relieved with premedication and following operation. Significant correlations were noted after premedication between observer and patient self-rating scores for apprehension and excitement.

The most sensitive self-rating index of drug effect was the 100 mm horizontal linear analogue scale for relaxation. UK patients were asked to make a vertical mark across the horizontal line along the scale from 0 'less relaxed' to 100 'more relaxed' with a band labelled 'usual' between 45 and 55 mm. This modification suggested by Hindmarch 1980 (personal communication) normalizes the data and reduces multimodal peaks. Two-way analysis of variance of the patient self-rating scores showed a significant decrease in anxiety after premedication across the five groups. Changes in similar scores for relaxation and depression did not achieve significance.

Changes in psychomotor function were quantified by using the Leeds Psychomotor Testing Apparatus. (Enquiries to Leeds Psychomotor Services, 2 Acomb Court, Front Street, Acomb, York, YO2 3BJ.) For the choice reaction time tests, the patient sat comfortably holding the display board within easy reach of the preferred index finger with the elbow flexed. Lights above each of the six radial buttons were switched on in random fashion and the time delay between the presentation of the light and its cancellation noted. The motor component was also measured by the time delay between release of the finger from the central button and touching the appropriately lit radial button. The patient received 12 light presentations for practice followed by a further 12 presentations for recording total and motor choice reaction times.

For critical flicker fusion threshold determination, four light-emitting diodes were arranged one metre from the patient's eyes at the same horizontal level on the hospital bed table. The frequency of flicker was increased from 10 Hz to 50 Hz at 1 Hz per second, and decreased in similar fashion. The patient pressed a hand-held button when the lights either began to appear fused or flickering, and the frequency at which this occurred was noted by the observer. The whole cycle was repeated to obtain three critical flicker to fusion thresholds and three critical fusion to flicker thresholds.

Pre-operative medication with four active drugs and placebo did not prolong total and motor components of choice reaction time. However, two hours after operation, the total choice reaction time was significantly more impaired after lorazepam 2 mg than in the other drug groups, but at four hours there was no difference between the groups.

The greater sensitivity of critical flicker to fusion threshold when compared with critical fusion to flicker threshold measurement was confirmed by this study (Wernberg *et al.*, 1980). All five groups depressed the critical flicker to fusion threshold with premedication and during recovery from anaesthesia. Mean group values had not returned to baseline the next day unlike choice reaction time measurements. Lorazepam 2 mg again produced significant depression of critical flicker to fusion threshold two and four hours after operation and the next day ($P < 0.001$).

The intensity of anterograde amnesia was tested by patient recall of five randomized pictures shown 60 minutes after premedication when assessed the day after operation. Oxazepam and clobazam do not appear to have intrinsic amnesic properties unlike diazepam, lorazepam and flunitrazepam, at the dose levels studied.

As a further objective assessment of premedication, the anaesthetist recorded the effect of the pre-operative medication immediately before induction of anaesthesia. Several different anaesthetists were involved in the two studies as this part of the protocol could not be standardized. It is reassuring to note that the groups receiving active drugs had a better chance of a satisfactory effect than those receiving placebo.

Before operation in the Christchurch study, we showed that moderate dose flunitrazepam 1 mg significantly increased drowsiness, relieved apprehension and reduced excitement when compared with placebo one hour after premedication. Moderate dose lorazepam 2.5 mg also achieved significant changes for drowsiness and apprehension but not for excitement. Doubling these doses did not increase the effect.

Before operation in the UK study, diazepam 10 mg achieved significantly more drowsiness than clobazam 20 mg , oxazepam 30 mg or placebo. Signs of decreased apprehension were apparent in the four active drug groups and following placebo.

Drowsiness the day after operation was shown to be significant in all the groups in the New Zealand study with the greatest effect from lorazepam 2.5 mg and 5.0 mg. This drowsiness was also evident in the early recovery period two and four hours after operation following lorazepam 2 mg premedication in the UK study. Psychomotor performance was also impaired in the early recovery period by lorazepam 2 mg with significantly increased choice reaction time two hours after operation.

Recall of events after premedication was significantly impaired with the greatest effect after flunitrazepam 2 mg and less after lorazepam 5 mg, flunitrazepam 1 mg and diazepam 20 mg in the first study. Lorazepam 2 mg achieved the greatest effect in the second study.

Dizziness and drowsiness were minimal following flunitrazepam 1 mg and this drug at this dose level offers better sedation and relief of anxiety without prolonged effect than diazepam 10 mg, lorazepam 2.5 mg or placebo for routine oral premedication in minor gynaecological surgery. Lorazepam 2 mg delayed early recovery and was therefore not suitable for premedication in day case surgery. Diazepam 10 mg gave more drowsiness than other benzodiazepines without active metabolites but did not delay early recovery. Amnesia for unpleasant aspects of the peri-operative period is a useful ingredient of premedication. Lack of recall of picture cards does not mean that the patient will not remember events such as the journey to the operating theatre and induction of anaesthesia, but recall of the long time spent lying on an uncomfortable theatre trolley may be obtunded.

Anxiety in Day Surgery Patients

Oral benzodiazepines have been shown to impair recovery following general anaesthesia for minor gynaecological surgery. A questionnaire survey of anxiety in day surgery patients was conducted to determine their suitability for a trial of new short-acting benzodiazepines for oral premedication (Male, 1981).

Patients were invited to mark a 100 mm horizontal line between the limits of 'calm' and 'terrified' to describe how they felt about the operation at that moment. Coincidentally and independently, a nurse noted the patients' anxiety as absent, slight, moderate or marked. Anxiety was assessed on admission, in the anaesthetic room and on discharge. When leaving the unit, the patients were asked if they would have liked a tablet before the operation to 'ease their nerves'.

A total of 118 patients (age 17–80 years) admitted consecutively to the day surgery unit were studied. There were 65 female and 53 male patients. Sixty-five operations were performed under local, and 53 under general anaesthesia. Most of the patients studied did not admit to, or show, much anxiety and only 17 of the 115 patients would have liked a tablet before the operation to 'ease their nerves'. Significantly more ($P < 0.02$) patients underwent local rather than general anaesthesia in this group. Patients who expressed a wish for oral anxiolytic premedication gave significantly higher ($P < 0.001$) anxiety scores on admission.

Day surgery patients undergoing local anaesthesia experienced significantly more anxiety after operation and may benefit from oral anxiolytic premedication.

The 100 mm linear analogue self-rating scale for patient anxiety proved more sensitive than the nurses' objective four-point assessment, but the choice of indices might be improved to give a more normal distribution.

From these results, we conclude that the variable characteristics of this population of day surgery patients, their ambivalence to anxiolytic oral premedication and the general low levels of anxiety documented, do not offer favourable conditions for a trial of short-acting benzodiazepines for oral premedication.

References

Dundee JW, Moore J and Nicholls RM (1962) Studies of drugs given before anaesthesia. I: A method of pre-operative assessment. *Br. J. Anaesth.*, **34**, 458.

Male CG, Lim YT, Male M, Stewart JM and Gibbs JM (1980) Comparison for three benzodiazepines for oral premedication in minor gynaecological surgery. *Br. J. Anaesth.*, **42**, 429–36.

Male CG (1981) Anxiety in day surgery patients. *Br. J. Anaesth.*, **53**, 663.

Male CG and Johnson HD (1984) Oral benzodiazepine premedication in minor gynaecological surgery. *Br. J. Anaesth.*, **56**, 499–507.

Wernberg M, Nielson SF and Hommelgaard P (1980) A comparison between reaction time measurement and critical flicker fusion frequency under rising nitrous oxide inhalation in healthy subjects. *Acta Anaesthesiol. Scand.*, **24**, 86.

Zuckerman M (1960) The development of an affect adjective check list for the measurement of anxiety. *J. Consult. Clin. Psychol.*, **24**, 457.

Aspects of Recovery from Anaesthesia
Edited by I. Hindmarch, J. G. Jones and E. Moss
© 1987 John Wiley & Sons Ltd

12

Assessment of Memory for Anaesthesia

K. Millar

University of Glasgow, Glasgow

Summary

Memory for anaesthesia is shown to be a well-substantiated phenomenon which is amenable to experimental investigation. The discussion concentrates upon two issues: the techniques for assessing memory for intra-operative events, and those factors which may modify the occurrence and detection of the phenomenon.

Introduction

It is well documented that some patients retain a memory of conversations and events that occurred while they were ostensibly unconscious during general anaesthesia (Mainzer, 1979; Mostert, 1975). Such memories may be extremely variable in nature, ranging from verbatim recall of conversations, through less distinct memories elicited by cueing techniques, to those subconscious memories which are evoked only when the patient is subject to hypnosis. The purpose of this chapter is to discuss a number of frequently neglected factors which may influence the sensitivity of assessment of intra-operative memory. It is likely that a proportion of memories go undetected for lack of such suitable assessment.

The chapter is divided into two main sections: discussion of the assessment of memory for anaesthesia, and the consideration of factors that may modify storage of material during anaesthesia.

Memory and Awareness as Linked Phenomena

It is quite often assumed that intra-operative memories are a consequence of periods of 'awareness' when the patient has been allowed inadvertently to enter a very light plane of anaesthesia. Certain anaesthetic techniques have been associated with greater likelihood of awareness (Breckenridge and Aitkenhead, 1983) whose detection may be made difficult by the use of muscle relaxants and premedicative agents which eliminate clinical signs of the level of anaesthesia. Thus, as in the case of memory for anaesthesia, the detection of awareness is critically dependent upon the sensitivity of the assessment technique.

While the present concern is with memory assessment, the concept of awareness is not irrelevant. The phenomena are linked: one must assume that memory is dependent on some degree of arousal or sensitivity to input in the unconscious patient.

However, the empirical evidence on this point seems contradictory: for example Tunstall (1977), using the isolated forearm technique (IFT), found intra-operative awareness in more than 75% of his patients but no subsequent recall of events. (The IFT involves inflating a blood pressure cuff around the arm to cut off the blood supply, hence preventing muscle relaxants from circulation in, and paralysing the arm. The patient can then make signals with the hand, either in response to command, or if spontaneously aware during surgery.)

Russell (1986) reported recall by only one patient in his sample of 25 although 11 showed movements in response to command and 18 made purposeful movements of the isolated arm. Conversely, Millar and Watkinson (1983), also using the IFT, found no evidence of awareness but significant recall of information. The methodological differences between the studies make it impossible to determine the basis of the discrepancy but one can recruit evidence from two other areas of experimentation to help resolve the issue.

Breckenridge and Aitkenhead (1983) and Jones and Koniezko (1986) have indicated the value of auditory evoked responses (ER) as indices of the depth of anaesthesia, and hence vulnerability to awareness. As it is well established that analysis of complex verbal input is a cortical function, it is important to note that while some anaesthetics spare the brain stem component of the auditory ER, there is reported to be a universal depressant effect upon the cortical component (Jones and Koniezko, 1986). The latter component is completely suppressed at doses equivalent to the MAC value. Thus, as Jones and Koniezko (1986) point out, certain anaesthetic concentrations will block the possible memorization of verbal material.

From the above, one can therefore conclude that memory for events may occur only at anaesthetic concentrations that permit some cortical registration of input. Although cortical suppression may be present at such concentrations, there is the possibility that auditory information may induce transient weak arousal—or co-occur with a spontaneous weak arousal—and be processed and stored at a subconscious level.

The latter hypothesis is somewhat speculative and requires support from empirical findings. Unfortunately, studies of EEG activity during learning in conscious subjects provide relatively little useful evidence on this point because the level of arousal during the input of information is modified by motivational and attentional factors that may not be present in anaesthetized subjects (Jones and Rhodes, 1978; Jones *et al.*, 1979a). Nonetheless, one should note that psychological performance studies of subliminal perception indicate extremely efficient subconscious processing and storage of information in conscious subjects (Dixon, 1981; Jacoby and Witherspoon, 1982). Such processing can be to a complex level of analysis indicating an access to higher cognitive processes without conscious awareness.

Evidence from studies of sleeping subjects may have greater bearing upon the issue. Early studies of learning during sleep (hypnopaedia) gave highly positive results. However, it was impossible to establish whether learning actually occurred during sleep or brief periods of wakefulness because no EEG measures were made of the sleep stage during learning (Bonnett, 1982). More recent EEG studies of sleep learning have established that some degree of arousal is necessary for learning to occur. Recall tends to be no better than chance unless 5–10 seconds of alpha activity occurs coincident with presentation of auditory information (Bonnet, 1982). Similarly, quite complex stimulus discriminations between meaningful sounds are possible during sleep but these are accomplished in the earlier sleep stages. Bonnet (1982) also points out that the use of financial incentives can significantly increase the number of successful discriminations made by sleeping subjects. The result implies that even in unconscious subjects 'higher cortical control can override reticular deactivation' (Bonnet, 1982).

From the discussion above, it seems reasonable to conclude that some degree of arousal will be necessary for learning to occur under anaesthesia. It is also evident that complex subconscious processing of input is possible without awareness when the individual is in a state of low arousal. Equally, if learning does occur under these conditions, the registration of input may be faint and the subsequent storage may be fragile. The sensitivity of the memory test will then be crucial to the detection of the stored material. In this regard, it may be useful to generalize from evidence presented by Brown *et al.* (1982) concerning the similarity between the amnesic state induced by certain drugs in normal subjects, and the memory impairment suffered by patients having organic amnesia. One might draw a further analogy between the patient who has retained information from anaesthesia and the organic amnesic patient; both groups of patients may have grossly defective retrieval if asked to give spontaneous recall of past events. However, the use of subtle cueing techniques often retrieves information from the memory of amnesic patients that would otherwise remain inaccessible. The surgical patient may show similar receptivity to a more subtle assessment. As will be seen below, relatively few studies have pursued such a hypothesis.

Experimental Studies of Retrieval

Free recall

Experimental studies of memory for anaesthesia have tended to follow a standard approach. Words or other auditory stimuli are presented during anaesthesia, sometimes with a concurrent attempt to detect periods of consciousness. On recovery, the patient is required to recall any events that occurred during anaesthesia.

Most of the studies that have used such a routine have found either that patients have no recall or that very faint recall is present in only a few patients (Eisele *et al.*, 1976; McIntyre, 1966; Brice *et al.*, 1970; Terrell *et al.*, 1969).

Millar and Watkinson (1983) and Millar (1983) have pointed out that the free recall routine probably underestimates the presence of material in memory. The task of free recall of information from memory places greater demands upon patients retrieval processes than do the tasks of cued recall and recognition (see Gregg, 1986). Amnesic patients tend to perform badly on free recall tasks but can show relatively less impairment with cued recall and certain aspects of recognition (see Eysenck, 1984; Jacoby and Witherspoon, 1982; Meudell and Mayes, 1984). If one pursues the analogy between the fragile retrieval state of amnesic patients and that of anaesthetized patients who have been exposed to information while unconscious, then tasks of cued recall and recognition may be more sensitive in detecting memory for anaesthesia. As will be shown below, there seems evidence to support this hypothesis.

Cued recall and recognition

Eysenck (1984) has cautioned against making sweeping generalizations about recall and recognition processes. The present review is, of necessity, brief and some generalization is inevitable: the reader should therefore consult Eysenck's text, and that of Gregg (1986) for a comprehensive view of the issue.

In cued recall, the retrieval of a word list may be prompted by the use of suitable cues; for instance the first letters of the words in the list or the names of the semantic categories to which the words belong. In the case of recognition, the patient is presented with a list of words and then, after an interval, is shown a test list consisting of the original words interspersed randomly amongst non-presented words. The patient must decide which words occurred in the original list. In the recognition task, the presence of the original words in the test list serves as cues to their location in memory. Such a cue may be of particular importance if the information has been weakly registered in a semi-conscious state (Millar and Watkinson, 1983). In other words, recognition may provide the patient with the opportunity to take advantage of only partial learning of the material (Baddeley, 1976).

Dubovsky and Trustman (1976) employed a recognition task to examine memory in anaesthetized obstetric patients. Patients were presented with letter-word pairs (e.g. 'G' is for 'Game' etc.) and their ability to recognize the original pairings was tested when recovered. Patients who had been presented with the original pairings did not differ from a control group in their chance ability to choose the correct pairs. However, the negative result is uncertain for two reasons. First, Dubovsky and Trustman (1976) make no assessment of awareness during word presentation. It is therefore quite possible that the depth of anaesthesia simply made it unlikely that any information would be registered. Secondly, the authors expressed recognition performance only in terms of the number of correct responses. But a further important dimension of performance is the 'false alarm rate' where patients chose pairings which were not presented during anaesthesia. Experimental and control groups might make similar numbers of correct detections but differ in their false alarms, the latter perhaps implying a difference in the propensity to guess or, more importantly, in their discriminative ability. The correct detection and false alarm rates can be transformed mathematically by Signal Detection Theory (Egan, 1975; McNicoll 1972) to describe recognition in terms of the two parameters d' (pronounced 'd-prime') and beta. The parameter d' is a numerical index of the patient's ability to discriminate between presented and non-presented words. Beta indicates the degree of caution in the discriminative decision process. The analysis has been widely used in memory research and adds considerable sensitivity to the assessment.

Millar and Watkinson (1983) extended Dubovsky and Trustman's (1976) research by employing a signal detection analysis of recognition performance in 53 obstetric patients. Twenty-seven patients were presented with lists of 10 words while anaesthetized; the remaining 26 control patients heard a tape of radio static. Awareness was assessed by the IFT (Tunstall, 1977). Millar and Watkinson found no reliable evidence of awareness in their control or experimental groups and no patient had any spontaneous recall of intra-operative events. Analysis of simple correct recognition performance revealed no significant difference between the groups. However, when the data were transformed to the values d' and beta, the experimental group showed significantly better performance in discriminating between presented and non-presented words on the recognition test (Figure 1). The groups did not differ significantly in their beta values, but the experimental group did show overall higher scores indicating greater caution in the decision process.

The results of Millar and Watkinson (1983) confirm a number of points about retrieval tasks and their application to intra-anaesthetic memory. First, spontaneous recall from memory is not a reliable indicator of whether or not information has been retained from the anaesthetic period. Secondly, a

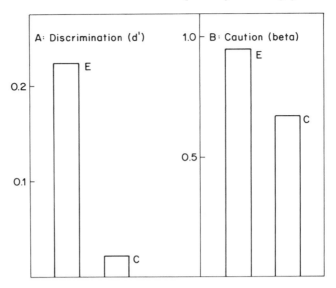

Figure 1. Panel A shows the average discrimination scores of the experimental (E) and control (C) patients. Panel B shows the degree of caution applied by the groups in their discrimination decision.

recognition test requires sophisticated analysis involving all performance parameters, if a sensitive assessment is to be made. A recent negative finding reported by Eich *et al.* (1985) in a study of recognition following anaesthesia may be due to failure to make such an analysis. Correct detection and false alarm rates were not transformed to signal detection parameters. The authors also failed to make any assessment of awareness or to give sufficient details of the anaesthetic. It is possible that their patients were so deeply anaesthetized as to preclude any storage of events (see Bennett and Boyle, 1986 for discussion of other difficulties in the research of Eich *et al.*, 1985).

Finally, given that the previous discussion suggested some degree of arousal is necessary for information to be stored in memory during anaesthesia, it might appear from Millar and Watkinson's (1983) results that the IFT may be insensitive to some states of arousal. While difficulties with the IFT have been outlined by other authors (Russell, 1979, 1981; Clapham, 1981), one should note Millar and Watkinson's observation that their patients did produce more arm movements during intubation and at the moment of the first incision. Such movements would suggest some sensitivity to noxious stimulation which, in turn, might imply some awareness of events.

Anaesthesia and Subsequent Behaviour Change

Non-verbal response to intra-operative events

It can be argued that while traditional experimental studies of memory for anaesthesia help to determine the circumstances and tasks that are most likely to define the phenomenon, they have little real life or 'ecological' validity. Consequently, there is perhaps more practical merit in establishing whether intra-operative events have a subconscious or conscious consequence for later waking thoughts and behaviour. Such an approach has been taken by Bennett *et al.* (1985) in an interesting study of non-verbal response to intra-operative conversation. Their study is worth considering in moderate detail because it reveals a number of important methodological and logical difficulties which unfortunately obscure interpretation of the results.

While anaesthetized, 11 experimental patients were presented with the tape recorded suggestion that in a post-operative interview they would pull their ear to indicate that they had heard the intra-operative message. A control group of 22 patients heard operating room sounds. Subsequently, no patient had any conscious recall of intra-operative events, but the experimental patients were reported to be significantly more likely to touch their ear during the post-operative interview and to spend a longer time ear-pulling.

The primary difficulty with the results concerns the omission of a pre-surgical assessment of 'ear-pulling' in order to determine the baseline frequency of the behaviour.

Without such a baseline, one cannot determine unequivocally whether the post-surgical difference between the groups is due to the intra-anaesthetic suggestion or to chance allocation to the experimental group of patients with a naturally higher frequency of the behaviour. With such small sample sizes and the biased allocation of patients to groups (2:1; control versus experimental), the latter probability is high.

The second difficulty stems directly from the small size of the experimental group where extreme reactions by one or two patients may give a misleading result. This is well illustrated by two patients in the experimental group who each spent 300 sec pulling their ears, accounting between them for 600 of the total 667 sec spent ear-pulling by the 11 members of the group. These same two patients also accounted for 29 of the 66 separate ear-pulls made by the experimental group. If the latter two patients were excluded from the analysis it is unlikely that the groups would differ significantly (see Figure 2 which displays the original and revised data of Bennett *et al.*, 1985).

Finally, an anaesthetized patient, within whose presence a surgeon made pessimistic comments about the bone graft being performed, took longer to recover and required more analgesia than other patients. The authors imply that the comments exerted a subconscious influence upon recovery. However,

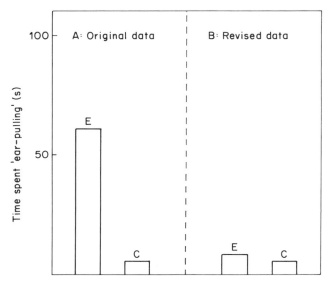

Figure 2. Panel A shows the original data presented by Bennett *et al*. (1983). Panel B shows the revised data form as described in the present text. Both panels show the time spent 'ear-pulling' in the post-operative interview. E = experimental group, C = control group.

given the surgeon's objective assessment of the unsatisfactory surgical procedure, it is surely more parsimonious to conclude that the patient's extended and painful recovery was due to physical discomfort arising from imperfect surgery rather than subconscious trauma.

Changes in dynamics of verbal memory

An alternative approach to examining the more practical aspects of memory is to consider changes in the dynamics of the memory system following exposure to intra-operative information. As many patterns of thought and behaviour depend critically upon the retrieval of information stored in memory, any intra-operative influence upon memory could have far-reaching consequences.

Verbal material can usefully be conceptualized as having a hierarchical organization within the human semantic memory system (that part of memory concerned with the meaning of words and their inter-relationships). Thus words which have a semantic relationship (e.g. dog, horse, ocelot) can be conceptualized as lying at different levels in the hierarchy of their common category (all four-legged animals). The frequency of a word in the language tends to determine its position in the hierarchy which, in turn, determines the probability of its recall when an individual is asked to free associate to a particular category name (see Freedman and Loftus, 1971; Gregg, 1986).

It is known that the order and nature of words recalled from given categories show similarity from one individual to another, reflecting the common language usage within the population (Battig and Montague, 1969). Moreover, and crucially from the present point of view, exposure to words in a particular category not only increases the probability that they will subsequently be retrieved, but also makes it more likely that those words will be recalled earlier in the retrieval sequence than if such priming had not taken place. In other words, exposure to a word tends to raise its level or 'dominance' in the hierarchy.

Given the above, one would predict that if anaesthetized patients are capable of registering information during anaesthesia which will have effects upon their subsequent verbal behaviour, then when they are presented intra-operatively with a list of semantically related words, the profile of their subsequent free retrieval from that semantic category may be changed.

The hypothesis has been tested by the present author and his colleagues with a group of patients undergoing brief obstetric and gynaecological procedures. Six tape-recorded lists of eight words were prepared. Each list was assigned a different semantic category (e.g. flowers, animals, etc.) such that, within a list, the words were all moderately common examples of that category. Patients were allocated at random to one of the lists which was repeated during anaesthesia.

Some hours after recovery, patients were asked to free associate to all six of the word lists (no patient had any recall of the intra-operative events). Figure 3 shows the probability of recalling a list word within the first 10 words given as free associates to the category names. The shaded histogram represents recall of words from lists which were presented during anaesthesia. The open histogram shows the patients' spontaneous production of words in the other five lists which were not presented to them. As Figure 3 reveals, words in the lists presented during anaesthesia were more likely to be recalled earlier in the retrieval sequence, suggesting that prior exposure to the words raised their priority for retrieval. The difference in the recall profiles is significant ($P < 0.01$).

The result is an interesting illustration of the subconscious influence of intra-anaesthetic information upon subsequent verbal behaviour. The dynamics of the semantic memory system have been altered so as to bias patients towards retrieval of a particular class of information. One might cautiously generalize from this result to suggest that other neutral, or emotionally coloured, auditory information heard during anaesthesia may have a similar effect. Indeed, studies of retrieval under hypnosis, described below, provide quite strong influence for the impact of emotional material.

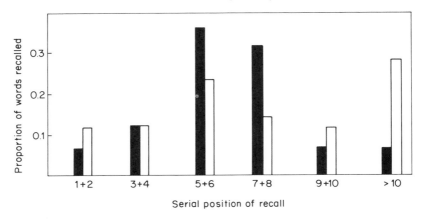

Figure 3. The proportion of words freely recalled from semantic categories as a function of presentation (shaded bars) and non-presentation (open bars) during anaesthesia.

Hypnosis and recall

Some authors suggest that very disquieting information may be repressed from consciousness such that it can be accessed only by hypnosis. As disquieting information may be 'heard' during anaesthesia concerning a pessimistic diagnosis or prognosis, it has been proposed that psychological disturbances can arise, and their basis may go unrecognized unless the patient is subject to questioning under hypnosis (Cheek, 1964; Blacher, 1975). Cheek (1959) provides an interesting series of case histories which illustrate hypnotic retrieval of traumatic events during surgery which were inaccessible to conscious recall by patients.

Levinson (1965) has provided experimental evidence for subconscious storage of traumatic events during surgery. While patients were anaesthetized and undergoing surgery, Levinson fabricated anaesthetic crises, making statements such as 'the patient is turning blue' and reading out dire diagnoses such as 'the lung looks cancerous' (reported by Mostert, 1975).

Of the 10 patients studied under hypnosis, four could recall the events and information that occurred. Two patients became so distressed as to awake from the hypnotic trance.

Levinson's results provide quite powerful evidence for the subconscious registration of traumatic events during surgery. However, as it is unlikely that any present-day ethical committee would permit an attempt to replicate Levinson's study, it may be difficult to examine further the impact of traumatic information upon memory during anaesthesia in any systematic way. Interpretation of the results of more opportunistic observations, such as those of Bennett *et al*. (1985) described above, are not without difficulties (see Millar, 1986).

The more general issue of the role of hypnosis as a retrieval aid has perhaps suffered adverse media attention, particularly in the light of claims that individuals may be regressed to memories of previous existences. If retrieval of such memories is possible, then retrieval of information from a period of anaesthesia would seem a rather minor achievement! However, the more fantastic claims do illustrate the point that hypnotic recall can be embellished with confabulation and exaggeration, and that hypnosis can make subjects less cautious of the material they relate (see Gregg, 1986). Equally, investigators who are not 'blind' to the information which the subject should be recalling, may be more lax in their criterion for accepting retrieved material representative of that information. Conversely, where no objective record is available of events that occurred during anaesthesia, it may be impossible to verify a patient's recall. Moreover, patients may confuse memory for events occurring peri-operatively and attribute them to the anaesthetic period.

Overall, therefore, one might question whether a hypnotic recall technique can be applied with sufficient rigour to provide reliable data.

From the above considerations of some techniques for assessing recall, one might conclude that further experimentation will benefit from the use of retrieval tasks derived from well-established findings of experimental psychology. Such tasks have the potential to provide an unambiguous measure of retrieval and the sensitivity to probe within memory for faintly registered material that would remain inaccessible to spontaneous recall.

Factors Modifying Memory for Anaesthesia

The modifying influence of the anaesthetic concentration upon memory storage has been considered in an early section of this paper. Four other factors are worth considering.

Premedication and amnesia

It is often argued that some premedicative drugs employed prior to surgery exert an amnesic influence that may depress the registration and recall of material presented during anaesthesia. While drugs such as diazepam, lorazepam and hyoscine can impair memory performance, it is quite incorrect to regard them as having a general amnesic effect.

First, Jones *et al*. (1978) showed that while diazepam and hyoscine both impaired short-term memory performance, neither drug had any adverse effect upon the recall of categorizable lists of words (words having semantic relationships). As the latter meaningful information is more similar to the information to which a patient may be exposed during anaesthesia, the result implies that premedicative drugs might have no amnesic influence upon it. Similarly, Ghoneim *et al*. (1984) found dose-related impairment of short-term memory by diazepam, but no effect upon the probability of retrieval on a long-term semantic recognition task. The speed with which words were generated from semantic memory was impaired by diazepam, but Millar *et al*. (1980) have shown that response speed cannot be taken to reflect retrieval processes per se. Mewaldt *et al*. (1986) have recently shown similar lack of impairment of semantic memory by diazepam. More generally, File and Lister (1982) have provided evidence that may suggest it is the non-specific sedative effect of lorazepam that effects memory performance rather than the processes of memory per se.

Two rather more extreme findings should be noted. Eisele *et al*. (1976) found no evidence of amnesia following a range of premedicative drugs. They suggest either that the drugs have no amnesic effect or that their effects are so transient as to have no intra-operative consequence. One might also note Turner and Wilson's (1969) report that diazepam increased the frequency of unpleasant recall. While these results run counter to other evidence, they emphasize that administration of a premedicative drug is no guarantee that amnesia will occur for intra-operative events.

Individual differences

Claridge (1971) has shown that particular personality characteristics indicative of certain states of CNS arousal are more highly correlated with the amount of anaesthetic required to induce sedation than is the conventional criterion of body weight. Claridge concludes that body weight is a 'poor guide as to the dosage of drug required to sedate the individual' (Claridge, 1971). The implications of this finding is that for two individuals of equal weight but different CNS reactivity, the more highly aroused individual might be relatively less sedated by anaesthesia with obvious consequences for awareness and memory (see also Claridge *et al*., 1981).

Individual differences between patients may also modify the amnesic influence of a premedicative drug. Brown *et al*. (1983) found that only a sub-group of their experimental sample showed any consistent impairment of memory in response to lorazepam. The only influence of the drug upon retrieval from long-term semantic memory was in terms of the rate at which words were generated from memory; the probability of retrieval was not affected.

The importance of individual differences is further emphasized by Desai *et al*. (1983) who showed radically different effects of diazepam as a function of the chronic anxiety level of the patient. While low anxiety patients showed the 'conventional' impairment of short-term memory, the memory of highly anxious subjects was significantly improved by diazepam.

Such results not only cast doubt upon the notion of a general amnesic influence of diazepam and its consequences for intra-operative memory, but also create difficulties for those who attempt to develop theories of diazepam action upon memory without regard to the influence of individual factors (e.g. Mewaldt *et al.*, 1983).

State-dependent learning

State-dependent learning refers to the phenomenon whereby information is retrieved more readily when the CNS state is similar to that during learning. For instance, if one learns while sedated by a drug, one's retrieval of the information may tend to be superior when again sedated rather than in a 'normal' state (see Eich, 1980).

Dubovsky and Trustman (1976) have suggested that retrieval of intra-operative information is impaired because of the dissonance between the sedated state during learning and the fully conscious state at recall. Implicit here is the hypothesis that patients would recall intra-operative events if subjected once again to anaesthesia. However, as Millar and Watkinson (1983) have pointed out, quite how memory would be tested in unconscious patients remains unspecified!

Nonetheless, one should note that Adam *et al.* (1974) have shown state-dependent learning in volunteers inhaling isoflurane at levels that permitted retention of consciousness. When in an undrugged state, subjects could not recognize material which had been presented during inhalation, but on reinstatement of the drug the amnesia was removed.

Clearly, therefore, one should not be too dismissive of Dubovsky and Trustman's (1976) hypothesis. It seems entirely possible that information may be stored during anaesthesia which cannot be accessed due to the incompatibility of the states of learning and retrieval.

Circadian effects

The efficiency of learning and retrieval varies with changes in physiological arousal through the day (Baddeley *et al.*, 1970; Folkard and Monk, 1980; Millar *et al.*, 1980). Recall tends to be better for material learned early in the day when arousal is relatively low. Interestingly, in a re-analysis of Millar and Watkinson's (1983) data, patients in the experimental group who had anaesthesia in the morning showed significantly better recognition memory performance than those who had surgery in the afternoon. It is unlikely that the effect would be modified by an interaction between pre-medicative drugs and the circadian change in arousal because Ghoneim *et al.* (1984) report no circadian influence on the action of diazepam upon memory.

The result has implications both for general theory and anaesthetic practice. First, the result implies that circadian variation in memory efficiency is independent of conscious awareness or attentional factors. Secondly, patients having anaesthesia earlier in the day may be at a relatively greater risk of retaining auditory information.

Conclusions

It is evident that memory for anaesthesia is a real phenomenon. It is equally evident that detection of the phenomenon, and hence its apparent frequency of occurrence, may be modified by a number of factors. For instance, assessment routines applicable to amnesic patients have been shown to be more sensitive in detecting memory in surgical patients than straightforward measures of spontaneous recall.

However, one needs to consider very carefully just what might be the real practical value of the demonstration of retrieval by these measures. As a retrospective measure of awareness, it clearly has no value to the patient or anaesthetist as an indicator of possible consciousness at the moment it occurs during surgery (Millar, 1983). Rather, the importance of such memory research techniques probably will lie in conjunction with other tests of awareness in defining the levels of anaesthesia that will preclude any storage of experience. It has been noted above that cortical ER's permit one to relate certain levels of anaesthesia to activity within the CNS, and to determine the extent to which external events impinge upon the cortex. The parallel use of tests of memory may permit one to infer the degree to which such events, registered by the cortex, are likely to be stored in the long term. It may be that one will then be able to determine a relationship between the physical magnitude of the evoked sensory event permitted by a specified anaesthetic concentration, and the probability of retrieval.

But one would still require to be wary of too unsubtle an approach. This review has emphasized that the sensitivity of the assessment and analysis of memory performance is crucially important.

Many experimental studies have produced negative results. But, as has been shown, a number of factors can modify or mask the phenomenon, a few studies account for all of such factors. One should therefore be cautious in deciding whether a negative result has a reliable basis, or whether the results are simply a product of methodological omissions and insensitive analysis.

It has also been noted that unconscious processing may be to a high order of complexity; indeed sleeping subjects can be primed to react selectively to quite complex information in EEG-defined stage 4 sleep (Bonnet, 1982). Therefore, it may also be necessary to consider the emotional and semantic aspects of any stimulus material if one is to define precisely the arousal state and information conditions that will lead to recall. In this regard, it is relevant to note an observation that patients rarely recall trivial, non-significant information from an intra-anaesthetic episode (Cheek, 1959, 1964).

Ultimately, as Jones and Koniezko (1986) have suggested, such research may provide the anaesthetist with the ability to maintain anaesthesia at a concentration which apparently pre-empts memory, making the issue of awareness and memory for anaesthesia one of purely historical interest. That day may well come. However, for the moment, memory retains an enigmatic quality: it is the dilemma of the interrogator, working in a clinic or a prison cell, whether to accept the assurance by patients or prisoners that they can remember nothing, or to continue probing by subtle or unsubtle means to prise out that vestige of information that may be passively or wilfully withheld. At the moment, no-one can determine unequivocally whether or not a mind has retained a memory of an event; not even the owner of the mind itself.

References

Adam N, Castro AD and Clark DL (1974) State-dependent learning with a general anaesthetic (isoflurane) in man. *J. Life Sciences,* **4**, 125–34.

Baddeley AD (1976) *The Psychology of Memory.* New York: Basic Books.

Baddeley AD, Hatter JE, Scott D and Snashall A (1970) Memory and time of day. *Q. J. Exp. Psychol.,* **22**, 605–9.

Battig W and Montague WE (1969) Category norms for verbal items in 56 categories: a replication and extension of the Connecticut Category Norms. *J. Exp. Psychol.* Monograph, **80** (3, part 2).

Bennett HL and Boyle WA (1986) Selective remembering: anaesthesia and memory. *Anesth. Analg.,* **65**, 988–9.

Bennett HL, Davis HS and Giannini JA (1985) Non-verbal response to intra-operative conversation. *Br. J. Anaesth.,* **57**, 174–9.

Blacher RS (1975) On awakening paralysed during surgery. *JAMA.,* **234**, 67–8.

Bonnet M (1982) Performance during sleep. In Webb WB (ed.) *Biological Rhythms, Sleep and Performance.* New York: Wiley.

Breckenridge JL and Aitkenhead AR (1983) Awareness during anaesthesia. *Ann. R. Coll. Surg. Engl.,* **65**, 90–6.

Brice DD, Hetherington RR and Uting JE (1970) A simple study of awareness during anaesthesia. *Br. J. Anaesth.,* **42**, 535–42.

Brown J, Brown MM and Bowes JB (1983) Effects of lorazepam on rate of forgetting on retrieval from semantic memory and on manual dexterity. *Neuropsychologia,* **21**, 501–12.

Brown J, Lewis V, Brown M, Horn G and Bowes JB (1982) A comparison between transient amnesias induced by two drugs (diazepam and lorazepam) and amnesia of organic origin. *Neuropsychologia,* **20**, 55–70.

Cheek DB (1959) Unconscious perception of meaningful sounds during surgical anaesthesia as revealed under hypnosis. *Am. J. Clin. Hypn.,* **1**, 101–13.

Cheek DB (1964) Surgical memory and reaction to careless conversation. *Am. J. Clin. Hypn.,* **6**, 237.

Clapham MC (1981) The isolated forearm technique using pancuronium. *Br. J. Anaesth.,* **36**, 642.

Claridge GS (1971) The relative influence of weight and of 'nervous type' on the tolerance of amylobarbitone sodium. *Br. J. Anaesth.,* **43**, 1121–5.

Claridge GS, Donald JR and Birchall PMA (1981) Drug tolerance and personality. *Personality and Individual Differences,* **2**, 153–6.

Desai N, Taylor-Davies A and Barnett DB (1983) The effects of diazepam and oxprenolol on short-term memory in individuals of high and low state anxiety. *Br. J. Clin. Pharmacol.*, **15**, 197–202.

Dixon NF (1981) *Preconscious Processing*. Chichester: Wiley.

Dubovsky SL and Trustman R (1976) Absence of recall after general anaesthesia. *Anesth. Analg.*, **55**, 696–701.

Egan JP (1975) *Signal Detection Theory and ROC Analysis*. New York: Academic Press.

Eich E, Reeves JL and Katz RL (1985) Anaesthesia, awareness, and the memory/awareness distinction. *Anesth. Analg.*, **64**, 1143–8.

Eich JE (1980) The cue-dependent nature of state-dependent retrieval. *Memory and Cognition*, **8**, 157–73.

Eisele V, Weinreich A and Bartle S (1976) Perioperative awareness and recall. *Anesth. Analg.*, **55**, 513–8.

Eysenck MW (1984) *A Handbook of Cognitive Psychology*. London: Lawrence Erlbaum.

File SE and Lister RG (1982) Do lorazepam-induced deficits in learning result from impaired rehearsal, reduced motivation or increased sedation? *Br. J. Clin. Pharmocol.*, **14**, 545–50.

Folkard S and Monk TH (1980) Circadian rhythms in human memory. *Br. J. Psychol.*, **71**, 295–307.

Freedman JL and Loftus EF (1971) Retrieval of words from long-term memory. *J. Verb. Learn. Verb. Behav.*, **10**, 107–15.

Ghoneim MM, Hinrichs JV and Mewaldt SP (1984) Dose-response analysis of the behavioural effects of diazepam: 1. learning and memory. *Psychopharmacology*, **82**, 291–5.

Gregg VH (1986) *Introduction to Human Memory*. London: Routledge & Kegan Paul.

Jacoby LL and Witherspoon D (1982) Remembering without awareness. *Canadian Journal of Psychology*, **36**, 300–24.

Jones D, Gale A and Smallbone A (1979) Short-term recall of nine-digit strings and the EEG. *Br. J. Psychol.*, **70**, 97–119.

Jones DM, Jones MEL, Lewis MJ and Spritts TLB (1979) Drugs and human memory: effects of low doses of nitrazepam and hyoscine on retention. *Br. J. Clin. Pharmacol.*, **7**, 479–83.

Jones D and Rhodes R (1978) Short-term memory and the EEG: effects of instructions to rehearse. *Biol. Psychol.*, **7**, 239–48.

Jones JG and Koniezko K (1986) Hearing and memory in anaesthetised patients. *Br. Med. J.*, **292**, 1291–3.

Levinson BW (1965) States of awareness during general anaesthesia. *Br. J. Anaesth.*, **37**, 544–50.

McIntyre JWR (1966) Awareness during general anaesthesia; preliminary observations. *Can. Anaesth. Soc. J.*, **13**, 495–9.

McNicoll D (1972) *A Primer of Signal Detection Theory*. Sydney: Allen and Unwin.

Mainzer J (1979) Awareness, muscle relaxants and balanced anaesthesia. *Can. Anaesth. Soc. J.*, **26**, 386–93.

Meudell PR and Mayes AR (1984) Patterns of confidence loss in the cued recall of normal people with attentuated recognition memory; their relation to a similar amnesic phenomenon. *Neuropsychologia*, **22**, 41–54.

Mewaldt SP, Ghoneim MM and Hinrichs JV (1986) The behavioural actions of diazepam and oxazepam are similar. *Psychopharmacology*, **88**, 165–71.

Mewaldt SP, Hinrichs JV and Ghoneim MM (1983) Diazepam and memory: support for a duplex model of memory. *Memory and Cognition*, **11**, 557–64.

Millar K (1983) Awareness during anaesthesia. *Ann. R. Coll. Surg. Engl.*, **65**, 350–1.

Millar K (1986) Non-verbal response to intraoperative conversation—an artifact? Paper submitted for publication to *Br. J. Anaesth.*

Millar K, Styles BC and Wastell DG (1980) Time of day and retrieval from long-term memory. *Br. J. Psychol.* **71**, 407–14.

Millar K and Watkinson N (1983) Recognition of words presented during general anaesthesia. *Ergonomics*, **26**, 585–94.

Mostert JW (1975) States of awareness during general anaesthesia. *Perspect. Biol. Med.*, **19**, 68–76.

Russell IF (1979) Auditory perception under anaesthesia. *Anaesthesia*, **34**, 211.

Russell IF (1981) Letter to the Editor. *Br. Med. J.*, **280**, 1056.

Russell IF (1986) Balanced anaesthesia: does it anaesthetize? *Anesth. Analg.*, **64**, 941–2.

Terrell RK, Sweet WO, Gladfelter JH and Stephen CR (1969) Study of recall during anaesthesia. *Anesth. Analg.*, **48**, 86–90.

Tunstall ME (1977) Detecting wakefulness during general anaesthesia for Caesarean section. *Br. Med. J.*, **i**, 1321.

Turner DJ and Wilson J (1969) Effect of diazepam on awareness during Caesarean section. *Br. Med. J.*, **ii**, 736.

Aspects of Recovery from Anaesthesia
Edited by I. Hindmarch, J. G. Jones and E. Moss
© 1987 John Wiley & Sons Ltd

13

Day Case Anaesthesia and Memory. A Comparison of Methohexitone and Propofol

J. Noble

The General Infirmary, Leeds

Introduction

Rapid and complete recovery from anaesthesia is one of the primary objectives in anaesthesia for day case surgery and an essential part of recovery is the return of normal memory function (Ogg *et al*., 1979). Short-term memory may be regarded as the working memory, essential for normal cognitive activities, reasoning and judgement. Thus it is of the utmost importance that any new drug thought useful in anaesthesia for day surgery should not cause any significant impairment of memory from the time patients leave hospital.

Propofol (Diprivan) has been found a very promising addition to the armamentarium of the day case anaesthetist with respect to quality of anaesthesia and recovery as assessed clinically and using a number of psychometric tests (Baher *et al*., 1982; Mackenzie and Grant, 1985; Wells, 1985), at least rivalling other currently available drugs. However, the specific impairment of memory in an otherwise apparently recovered patient is a common occurrence post-operatively (Bethune, 1981) and some drugs such as benzodiazepines may be particularly potent amnesic agents (Subhan and Hindmarch, 1984), it is thus of importance to investigate propofol in this regard.

The assessment of delayed recall has been found a more sensitive means of measuring impaired short-term memory function after anaesthesia than immediate recall (Bethune, 1981). The Williams delayed recall test (Williams, 1968) has proved useful in the comparison of anaesthetic agents used in day surgery (Ogg *et al*., 1979, 1983; Kennedy and Ogg, 1985) leading to modifications in clinical practice. It was the aim of this study to investigate the

93

effect of propofol on post-operative memory function and compare this with methohexitone. Also a comparative assessment of short-term clinical recovery from anaesthesia was to be made.

Patients and Methods

Subjects and anaesthesia

Fifty healthy patients presenting for vaginal termination of pregnancy as outpatients were studied. Ages ranged from 16 to 36 years and all were ASA grade 1 as judged by outpatient screening questionnaire and assessment by the anaesthetist. Hospital Ethical Committee approval was obtained for the study and all patients gave informed consent to participate. Two groups of 20 patients were randomly allocated each to receive one of two anaesthetic techniques adminstered on a double-blind basis. Patients received alfentanil 7 μg/kg^{-1} intravenously followed after one minute by induction with either methohexitone 1.5 μg/kg^{-1} or propofol 2.5 μg/kg^{-1} intravenously. Anaesthesia was maintained with bolus doses of the same anaesthetic agent, 10–20% of induction dose, as required. Patients breathed 66% nitrous oxide in oxygen spontaneously via a mask and airway.

Premedicant drugs and oxytocics were not used. Ten patients awaiting the same surgical procedure and fulfilling the same inclusion criteria were studied pre-operatively as a control group.

Assessment of immediate recovery

Immediate clinical recovery was quantified using the Steward scoring system. Patients were assessed at one minute intervals after discontinuation of nitrous oxide by an observer unaware of the anaesthetic used. A score was awarded for consciousness, airway maintenance and spontaneous movement until a maximum was achieved, when the patient was considered recovered. Times taken to opening eyes on request and stating date of birth correctly were also recorded.

Assessment of delayed recovery

Short-term memory function was assessed using the Williams delayed recall test which has been described in detail elsewhere (Kennedy and Ogg, 1985; Bethune, 1981). Patients are shown a number of picture cards each of which bears line drawings of nine everyday objects. The objects are named by the investigator and the subjects are allowed one minute to memorize the card. After 10 minutes of distraction, in this case with another psychometric test, recall of the card is tested. Error scores are awarded for failure to recall objects spontaneously and after verbal and then visual prompting. Patients undergoing anaesthesia were tested pre-operatively and at one and two hours post-operatively. Patients in the control group were tested similarly but at half hourly intervals prior to their anaesthetics.

At each test, patients were shown two cards successively, one new card testing for new information, and one the same on each occasion, testing for retention of relatively older information gained pre-operatively. Performance is rated relative to baseline or pre-operative score, each patient acting as her own control. Memory function testing was carried out by an investigator unaware of treatment, except in the control group.

Statistical analysis

Demographic data and duration of anaesthesia and recovery times were compared between groups using Student's t test. Memory function was assessed within groups using the Wilcoxon signed rank sum test and between groups using the Wilcoxon rank sum test with chi square to increase sensitivity.

Results

Demographic and anaesthetic data

All three groups of patients were found to be statistically comparable in terms of age and weight (Table 1). The doses of hypnotic agents administered were comparable in terms of hypnotic potency. Duration of anaesthesia in patients receiving methohexitone and those receiving propofol was not significantly different.

Clinical recovery

Recovery from anaesthesia in the immediate post-operative period was the same for both methohexitone and propofol in terms of time taken to opening

Table 1. Demographic data, hypnotic agent dosage and total anaesthetic times for the three groups of patients (mean ± SEM)

Group	n	Age (yrs)	Weight (kg)	Dose of hypnotic (mg/kg)	Duration of anaesthesia (min)
Propofol	20	23.7 ± 1.9	57.0 ± 2.1	3.2 ± 0.1	9.5 ± 0.4
Methohexitone	20	22.3 ± 1.5	58.4 ± 1.2	2.8 ± 0.1	10.4 ± 0.5
Control	10	22.5 ± 2.1	61.5 ± 3.3	–	–

Table 2. Recovery data, times taken to a achievement of recovery criteria (mean ± SEM)

Group	Eyes opening (min)	Date of birth (min)	Maximum Steward score (min)
Propofol	5.8 ± 0.4	6.9 ± 0.4	7.5 ± 0.4
Methohexitone	6.4 ± 0.6	7.1 ± 0.6	8.2 ± 0.6

eyes on request (Table 2), stating date of birth correctly and time to fulfilment of Steward recovery criteria.

Post-operative memory function

New facts. In patients receiving either methohexitone or propofol, a significant impairment of memory for new information ($P < 0.05$) was found to be present when patients were tested one hour post-operatively (Table 3). This deficit had returned to pre-operative levels on testing at two hours post-operatively. No significant differences were found between the groups at either time (Table 4). The control group showed no impairment of memory for new facts at the corresponding testing times.

Old facts. Patients in both anaesthetic groups showed an improvement in memory for old information over baseline levels when tested one hour post-operatively (Table 5). This improvement was most marked (Table 6) in patients receiving methohexitone ($P < 0.01$). When tested at two hours post-operatively, this improvement was seen in both anaesthetic groups, that in patients receiving methohexitone being slightly more significant than propofol. Control patients showed an improvement in memory for old facts on equivalent testing times which was significant ($P < 0.05$) on the final test. No significant differences between the groups were noted at any of the times tested.

Table 3. 'New facts', postoperative error scores relative to baseline (mean ± SEM). A positive score represents an increase in errors

Group	1 hour postop	2 hour postop
Propofol	5.7 ± 2.7	1.0 ± 1.7
Methohexitone	6.1 ± 3.0	1.9 ± 2.0
Control	0.3 ± 2.1	0 ± 1.8

Table 4. 'New facts', statistical analysis of within group performance over preoperative levels and corresponding times in the control group using Wilcoxon signed rank sum test. Values between groups are not significantly different using Wilcoxon rank sum and chi square tests

Groups	N	Rank sum	P	N	Rank sum	P
		1 hour postop			2 hours postop	
Propofol vs 0	18	37.5	0.05	19	70	NS
Methohexitone vs 0	18	38	0.05	17	64.5	NS
Control vs 0	6	10	NS	7	4	NS

This reasserts the importance of issuing instructions for post-operative conduct, in the pre-operative period, and not placing reliance on orders given in the post-operative period, especially in the first two hours. Clearly, the issuing of supplementary written instructions to the patient would be helpful, and it is important that the person into whose care the patient is discharged must also be fully conversant with such instructions. It could also be argued that patients going home after day surgery should be constantly accompanied, as much as possible, in the following 24 hours. These considerations should also be applied to casualty and dental departments where it is not unusual for patients to leave hospital well within two hours of awaking from anaesthesia.

Patients in the control group, as might be expected, showed no real change in their ability to retain information for new facts. Their ability to retain information for older facts was no better than patients who had an intervening anaesthetic, especially those given methohexitone who showed a significant improvement on the second test not seen in controls. This is perhaps a little unexpected especially as the control patients were tested at shorter intervals than anaesthetized patients and this would tend to emphasize any learning effect, although patients in the control group may be more affected by

Table 5. 'Old facts', postoperative error scores relative to baseline (mean ± SEM). A negative score represents a decrease in errors

Group	1 hour postop	2 hours postop
Propofol	−0.7 ± 1.0	−2.3 ± 0.9
Methohexitone	−3.5 ± 1.0	−5.6 ± 1.7
Controls	−0.6 ± 1.8	−2.1 ± 0.9

Table 6. 'Old facts', statistical analysis of within group performance relative to preoperative levels and corresponding times in the control group using the Wilcoxon signed rank sum test. Values between groups are not significantly different using Wilcoxon rank sum and chi square tests

Groups	1 hour postop			2 hours postop		
	N	Rank sum	*P*	N	Rank sum	*P*
Propofol vs 0	12	28.8	NS	14	18.5	0.05
Methohexitone vs 0	13	4	0.01	14	5	0.01
Controls vs 0	6	10	NS	7	4	NS

pro-active inhibition (confusion with previously seen cards). Further, anaesthetized patients may be subject to compensatory effort (Millar, 1983) especially at the two hour testing time. These findings are consistent with previous observations that sedative drugs, even benzodiazepines (Clarke *et al*., 1970), can improve short-term recall if given shortly after the memory stimulus by preventing displacement with new input. Profound anterograde impairment for new information is still seen after the administration of these drugs.

Similar findings were obtained in the control group used by Kennedy and Ogg (1985) and were thought to be due to lack of commitment of the subjects awaiting their anaesthetics. Patients awaiting termination of pregnancy are generally very anxious and anxiety is known to adversely affect psychomotor performance (Hindmarch, 1980). Such pre-operative patients do not make very good comparisons with, albeit similar, post-operative patients whose 'ordeals' are over and often appear considerably more relaxed. Differences in memory performance have been found between in-patients and nurses used as control groups in a similar previous study (Ogg *et al*., 1983). The difficulty of finding a suitable control group, for psychomotor testing even of in-patients post-operatively (Scott *et al*., 1983), has been stressed before, controls tending to score worse than post-anaesthetic patients, probably because of institutionalization, an effect known to adversely affect psychomotor performance (Herbert, 1986). Unfortunately, it is impossible to give a 'placebo' anaesthetic. Ethical considerations would tend to preclude the use of a positive control in studies of outpatient anaesthesia although they are often used in psychological studies (Hindmarch, 1980) and may be suitable for in-patient studies. Patients undergoing surgery under local anaesthesia can be used where the surgery is appropriate, but psychomotor effects have been related to local analgesics (Kortilla, 1974). Careful selection, matching, rehearsal of subjects and the use of crossover trial designs is virtually impossible in the normal day surgery unit and still does not guarantee removal of treatment order effects (Millar, 1983). Where a direct comparison of two anaesthetic agents is to be made using established tests, it may be considered unnecessary to use a control group (Clayburn *et al.*, 1986; Moss *et al.*, 1986).

Many tests of psychomotor performance have been applied in the assessment of recovery from anaesthesia (Drummond, 1975; Herbert, 1978; Hindmarch, 1980) and are still being developed and refined (Salt *et al.*, 1985) as no perfect test seems yet to have been developed. It is generally accepted that complex 'real life' simulatory tests, such as car driving, are not necessary for the assessment of recovery (Herbert, 1978). Besides the practical difficulties involved, results can be confusing and no more meaningful than tests which measure some more restricted aspect of psychomotor function. Indeed apparent relevance, or face validity, of a test to the concept of street fitness is not an essential feature in such an assessment (Herbert, 1978), although if present it can be considered to give some additional relevance to findings. In general more physiologically esoteric tests, such as flicker fusion (Moss *et al.*, 1986) or reaction time testing (Wilkinson and Houghton, 1982) seem to be more sensitive to the effects of sedative drugs or drowsiness. The assessment of short-term memory has been considered one of the most useful means of measuring post-operative mental function (Drummond, 1975) and as outlined above has considerable face validity in the context of discharge from day surgery units. Many tests of memory performance have been utilized, including digit span, pictorial (iconic) recall and free recall of word lists. Williams (1968) found delayed recall for pictorial stimuli, the most sensitive of these tests in the detection of organic cerebral pathology. Similarly, Bethune (1980) found this test sensitive to organic amnesic states where deficits were not demonstrable using the digit span test and drew parallels with post-operative amnesia. Digit span was found unaffected by two outpatient anaesthetic techniques (Ogg *et al.*, 1979) one hour post-operatively when a highly significant deficit was found using the delayed recall test.

Subhan and Hindmarch (1984), however, found digit span sensitive to the amnesic effects of some benzodiazepine derivatives 19 hours after administration, thus it would be reasonable to regard the Williams delayed recall test as a potentially sensitive test of short-term memory function.

Each test of post-operative psychomotor function provides a balance (Drummond, 1975) of discrimination (recovered versus non-recovered patients) against sensitivity (the detection of residual drug activity). When patients are fit to leave the day surgery unit, they will almost certainly still have some residual drug activity with currently available agents, tests which are too sensitive would label them non-recovered and would not be of much assistance to the anaesthetist in his assessment of street fitness. The Williams delayed recall test may thus appear to be of adequate sensitivity for this purpose, but the detection of differences between methohexitone and propofol beyond the times studied in this chapter would require the use of more sensitive tests or perhaps greater numbers of patients. Critical flicker fusion frequency threshold (CFF) has been thought too sensitive for the assessment of recovery from day case anaesthesia (Grove-White and Kelman, 1971) although patients were only tested up to 90 minutes post-operatively. CFF has been found to detect abnormalities 12 hours after halothane anaesthesia in one study (Moss *et al.*, 1987) although no deficit was shown 30 minutes after anaesthesia with propofol and 60 minutes after methohexitone in another (Mackenzie and Grant, 1985) using similar test equipment. Choice reaction time was shown to be impaired eight hours after thiopentone anaesthesia (Scott *et al.*, 1983) and up to two days after halothane anaesthesia (Herbert *et al.*, 1983).

However, no deficit in choice reaction time could be demonstrated 30, 60 and 90 minutes after anaesthesia with propofol, methohexitone and thiopentone, respectively, in another study (Mackenzie and Grant, 1985). Whilst these apparently very sensitive tests seem to discriminate against thiopentone and halothane for day surgery, some confusion remains and they have not yet resolved the differences between methohexitone and propofol. Much more work obviously needs to be done, the simple unprepared reaction time test (Wilkinson and Houghton, 1982), a test of adult (Salt *et al.*, 1985) and paediatric visual perception threshold and a memory based reaction time test (HPRU, 1986) may prove additional tools for the further improvement and rationalization of anaesthesia for day surgery.

References

Bahar M, Dundee JW, O'Neill MP, Briggs, LP, Moore J and Merrett JD (1982) Recovery from intravenous anaesthesia. Comparison of disoprofol with thiopentone and methohexitone. *Anaesthesia*, **37**, 1171–5.

Bethune DW (1980) The assessment of brain damage following open-heart surgery. Proceedings of an international symposium. *Psychic and Neurological Dysfunctions after Open Heart Surgery*. Stuttgart: Georg Thieme Verlag, 100–6.

Bethune DW (1981) Test of delayed memory recall suitable for assessing post-operative amnesia. *Anaesthesia*, **34**, 942–8.

Clarke, PRF, Eccersley PS, Frisby JP and Thornton JA (1970) The amnesic effect of diazepam (Valium). *Br. J. Anaesth.*, **42**, 690–7.

Clayburn P, Kay NH and McKenzie PJ (1986) Effects of diazepam and midazolam on recovery from anaesthesia in outpatients. *Br. J. Anaesth.*, **58**, 872–5.

Drummond GB (1975) The assessment of post-operative mental function. *Br. J. Anaesth.*, **47**, 130–42.

Grove-White IG and Kelman GR (1971) Critical flicker fusion frequency after small doses of methohexitone, diazepam and 4 hydroxybutyrate. *Br. J. Anaesth.*, **43**, 110–2.

Herbert M (1978) Assessment of performance in studies of anaesthetic agents. *Br. J. Anaesth.*, **50**, 33–7.

Herbert M (1986) The duration of post-anaesthetic mental impairment. *Aspects of Recovery from Anaesthesia*. Proceedings of a symposium, York.

Herbert, M, Healy TEJ, Bourke JB, Fletcher IR and Rose JM (1983) Profile of recovery after general anaesthesia. *Br. Med. J.*, **286**, 1539–42.

Hindmarch I (1980) Psychomotor function and psychoactive drugs. *Br. J. Clin. Pharmacol.*, **10**, 189–209.

Human Psychopharmacology Research Unit (1986) Department of Psychology. University of Leeds, UK.

Kennedy DJ and Ogg TW (1985) Alfentanil and memory function. A comparison with fentanyl for day case termination of pregnancy. *Anaesthesia*, **40**, 537–40.

Kortilla E (1974) Psychomotor skills related to driving after intramuscular lidocaine. *Acta Anaesthesiol. Scand.*, **18**, 290–6.

Mackenzie N and Grant IS (1985) Comparison of the new emulsion formulation of propofol with methohexitone for day case anaesthesia. *Br. J. Anaesth.*, **57**, 725–31.

Millar K (1983) Clinical trial design: the neglected problem of asymmetrical transfer in cross over trials. *Psychol. Med.*, **13**, 867–73.

Moss E, Hindmarch I, Pain AJ and Edmonson RS (1987) A comparison of recovery after halothane or alfentanil anaesthesia for minor surgery. *Br. J. Anaesth.* **59**, 970–7.

Ogg TW, Fischer HBJ, Bethune DW and Collis JM (1979) Day case anaesthesia and memory. *Anaesthesia*, **34**, 784–9.

Ogg TW, Jennings RA and Morrison CG (1983) Day-case anaesthesia for termination of pregnancy. Evaluation of a total intravenous technique. *Anaesthesia*, **38**, 1042–6.

Scott WAC, Whitwam, JG and Wilkinson RT (1983) Choice reaction time. A method of measuring post-operative psychomotor performance decrements. *Anaesthesia*, **38**, 1162–8.

Salt PJ, Francis RI, Noble J and Ogg TW (1985) Assessment of recovery from anaesthesia using a new visual perception test. *Br. J. Anaesth.*, **57**, 820–1.

Subhan Z and Hindmarch I (1984) Assessing residual effects of benzodiazepines on short-term memory. *Pharm. Med.*, **1**, 27–32.

Wells JKG (1985) Comparison of ICI 35868, etomidate and methohexitone for day case anaesthesia. *Br. J. Anaesth.*, **57**, 732–5.

Wilkinson RT and Houghton D (1982) Field test of arousal. A portable reaction timer with data storage. *Human Factors*, **24**, 487–98.

Williams M (1968) The measurement of memory in clinical practice. *Br. J. Sociol. Clin. Psychol.*, **7**, 18–34.

Aspects of Recovery from Anaesthesia
Edited by I. Hindmarch, J. G. Jones and E. Moss
© 1987 John Wiley & Sons Ltd

14

The Duration of Post-anaesthetic Mental Impairment

M. Herbert

Nottingham University Medical School, Nottingham

Introduction

At a time of relatively slow economic growth and in the face of unrelenting demand for prompt and adequate health care, the health services in general are having to seek other ways to provide an effective service. In the field of surgery, one such way is to carry out relatively minor, elective procedures on a day case basis. This usually involves patients reporting directly to the day case unit where, after formal admission routines, they are prepared for surgery and the operation is carried out. After a brief recovery period during which patients regain consciousness, are able to carry out simple instructions and give adequate verbal responses to questions, they are discharged home into the care of a responsible adult, usually a family member.

As far as hospitals are concerned, day case units certainly appear to be cost-effective because hospital beds are not taken up by short-stay patients and other hotel facilities are perhaps being used more equitably. However, from the viewpoint of total patient care, the use of day case procedures carries special considerations having medico-legal connotations.

If the surgical procedure is a relatively minor one and if patients feel to be in no great discomfort they may well decide to resume their normal daily routine very soon after the operation. Indeed, Ogg (1972) discovered that 73% of car owners had driven within 24 hours of minor outpatient anaesthesia and that 9% had driven themselves home after surgery. Other hazardous routines could involve operating complex machinery or having to make rapid decisions.

These activities may be undertaken by patients who, very recently, had been rendered and kept unconscious by the administration of powerful CNS depressing drugs. The question therefore arises as to how long those drugs are likely to have measurable hangover effects and, in consequence, for how long patients should be advised to refrain from potentially dangerous acts such as car driving. Is it a reasonable assumption that if patients feel no after-effects and consider themselves to have made a full recovery that they are likely to be fit enough to resume daily life?

One way to approach such questions is to give patients recovering from anaesthesia various tests measuring psychomotor or other higher cortical functions. There are, of course, problems in extrapolating from the results of such tests to real life situations (Nicholson, 1976; Hindmarch, 1980), but it seems reasonable to assume that if particular abilities are impaired by psychoactive drugs, then everyday tasks calling upon those abilities are also likely to be adversely affected.

Short-term Studies of Recovery

A number of studies using a wide variety of anaesthetic agents, tests and subjects have concluded that the adverse mental effects of anaesthesia are relatively short-lived.

Hannington-Kiff (1970) used a Maddox Wing test to measure ocular divergence which is produced as a result of the generalized reduction in muscle tone caused by anaesthetic agents. Having tested unpremedicated dental outpatients, he reported that all patients anaesthetized with inhalational halothane, oxygen and nitrous oxide had returned to pre-operative levels of ocular divergence at 20 minutes after surgery. By 30 minutes after completion of dental extraction, 80% of patients who were induced into anaesthesia by methohexitone and 70% induced by propanidid had recovered to pre-operative levels.

Although the Maddox Wing test is unlikely to be a test of higher mental abilities, these results do suggest that the duration of action of some of the agents investigated may be relatively short. Hannington-Kiff went on to make the important point that tests of post-operative recovery should be sensitive enough to detect impairment which may not otherwise be clinically obvious.

A simple test which does appear to measure higher cortical functions and which also supports the idea of rapid post-anaesthetic recovery times was described by Sikh and Dhulia (1979). They asked unpremedicated patients undergoing minor orthopaedic procedures to add up the value of a number of coins of different denominations. It took patients induced into anaesthesia with thiopentone a total of 28 minutes to regain pre-operative speed and those receiving propanidid, a mean of 9.3 minutes.

One of the earliest reports to consider the use of performance tests in measuring recovery from anaesthesia was that by Vickers (1965). He asked volunteers to carry out a test of manual dexterity which involved transferring pegs from one set of holes to another. Again, using a return to pre-operative values as a criterion of recovery he concluded that even after his most potent combination of induction agent and dosage (thiopentone, 3 mg/kg), performance had returned to normal after 105–120 minutes. Using a modified version of the same test, Carson *et al*. (1975) found that 6 mg/kg of thiopentone delayed full recovery for about 35 minutes and that doubling the dose produced impairment lasting 90 minutes. Also using a measure of manual dexterity similar to the peg-board test, Sinclair and Cooper (1983) noted a rapid recovery to pre-anaesthetic levels of performance in unpremedicated female patients given alfentanil as a supplement to anaesthesia. On average, patients had recovered in about 25 minutes.

A number of studies have adopted the strategy of giving to people undergoing anaesthetic procedures, a battery of performance tests sampling a wide range of mental abilities. This approach is based on the notion that different agents or clinical techniques might differentially affect specific mental abilities. Gale (1976), for example, gave a total of 11 motor and cognitive tests ranging from reaction time tests to measures of arithmetic ability and colour naming skills. Despite this diversity of tests and varying combinations of anaesthetic regimens, most of the measures had returned to normal values by 2–3 hours post-operatively.

Korttila *et al*. (1977) used a battery of psychological tests measuring perceptual speed, manual dexterity, reaction time and measures derived from a car driving simulator. Healthy volunteers underwent an inhalational anaesthetic with either enflurane or halothane and their performance on the tests was measured at 2, 4, 5 and 7 hours after anaesthesia. Compared with an unanaesthetized control group tested at corresponding times, the experimental subjects performed significantly worse on the dexterity task and some aspects of the reaction time test up to 5 hours after anaesthesia. Impairment of driving skills was evident at 4.5 hours after halothane anaesthesia. The authors advised that patients given either of these two agents should not drive or operate machinery for at least 7 hours afterwards.

Other anaesthetic agents may produce even longer-lasting effects. In an extensive study of different induction agents on post-anaesthetic driving skills, Korttila *et al*. (1975) showed that, when compared with a control group, impairment was still evident 8 hours after induction of anaesthesia using thiopental or methohexital. Because of the severity of the disturbances of ability, the authors considered that patients given those agents should 'probably not drive for 24 hours', an opinion which was restated more strongly by Korttila (1981).

This opinion plus the fact that many studies report relatively brief impairment of mental abilities after anaesthesia appears to have had a strong influence on the advice which anaesthetists are prepared to give their patients. A recommendation by Havard (1976) that it is safer to advise patients against driving for 48 hours post-operatively was considered unnecessary by Baskett and Vickers (1979). They believed that an interval of 24 hours or a night's sleep would normally be regarded as sufficient.

Since the matter is of some importance it becomes necessary to look more closely at the evidence. Epstein (1975) pointed out that the literature describing recovery from anaesthesia was confusing and contradictory. Often data derived from healthy volunteers were compared with values from mixed-aged patients undergoing a variety of surgical procedures, and given varying doses of different anaesthetics.

It seems too that there are other methodological problems with several studies. Many tests of mental functioning are markedly susceptible to practice effects. People become more proficient or faster the more often they encounter the test, a point which Vickers (1965) had noticed when using his peg-board test. To compare several post-operative measures with one taken before anaesthesia is clearly going to confound drug-induced impairment of performance with improvement in efficiency due to practice. The resulting data would be biased towards demonstrating an artificially early recovery. To prevent this, patients either need to be practised to asymptote on the tests—a procedure which is usually not clinically feasible—or control groups are needed for comparison purposes.

Control groups, of course, should be tested not only at identical times to the experimental groups but also in identical circumstances. If patients are hospitalized after surgery it may be inappropriate to compare their performance with that of healthy, ambulatory control subjects since prolonged bed-rest alone can have detrimental effects on performance (Edwards *et al.*, 1981). Few studies report the times of day at which subjects are tested, but diurnal variation in psychological functioning whereby people generally improve their performance as the day goes on, is a well-recognized phenomenon (Hockey and Colquhoun, 1972) and needs to be carefully controlled.

Herbert (1978) drew attention to many variables which need to be considered when assessing the relationship between performance and anaesthetic agents, one of the most important of which is the question of test sensitivity. Not all tests are equally effective in detecting impairments which are not clinically obvious. In general terms a test becomes more sensitive the more familiar it is, the longer it lasts, the more it demands sustained output or maintained concentration and the less it is perceived as challenging or as novel and interesting. For such reasons, giving a battery of brief and unusual tests can be counter-productive. Subjects are likely to have their interest aroused by the procedures and, in consequence, residual impairment may be masked by increased motivation.

Many of the studies reporting relatively short-lived duration of post-anaesthetic mental impairment fall prey to one or more of these difficulties. However, two studies by MacKenzie and Grant (1975a; 1975b) overcome many of the problems which characterize research in this field. They investigated the post-anaesthetic sequelae of propofol, a relatively new anaesthetic drug, either for induction or for induction and maintenance of anaesthesia, in comparison with other anaesthetic agents in common use. Tests of critical flicker fusion threshold and choice reaction time were given pre-operatively and extended post-operatively to 120 minutes (1975a) and 240 minutes (1975b). A control group of patients matched for age, sex and weight were tested at identical times and under similar circumstances to the study groups and all patients were familiarized with the tests, to reduce practice effects.

Despite the inclusion of control patients, the authors elected not to make comparisons between them and the anaesthetic groups at the post-operative measurement points. Instead, each group was examined individually for post-operative impairment as compared with their own pre-operative baseline. It was concluded that following induction of anaesthesia by propofol, performance had recovered 60 minutes after. Impairment on some measures was still evident at 60 and 90 minutes following inductions by methohexitone and thiopentone respectively (1975a). The same method of analysis in the second study (1975b) revealed deficits in flicker fusion lasting up to 4 hours following induction and maintenance of anaesthesia with propofol.

Studies of immediate recovery from anaesthesia appear to be based on the assumption that once performance has returned to pre-anaesthetic levels, no further deterioration will take place. As a result, tests of mental abilities are usually not extended for longer than a few hours into the post-operative period. However, if performance is 'naturally' poorer at some times of day, patients may well be more vulnerable at such times to residual hangover effects and anaesthetic agents themselves may influence the normal circadian rhythms (Folkard *et al.*, 1979). The assumption of permanent recovery, once baseline levels of abilities have been achieved may be an unwise one to make.

Longer-term Studies of Recovery

A few studies have prolonged testing for more than one post-operative day. James (1969), for example, gave healthy volunteers a complex battery of tests for varying periods of time after cyclopropane anaesthesia and reported quite marked impairment of 'number facility' in the experimental group when compared with controls, two days after anaesthesia. Similarly, Riis *et al.* (1983) noted maximum deficits in attentional skills of elderly patients two days after surgery when compared with pre-operative baselines.

Davison *et al.* (1975), compared the performance of two groups anaesthetized for 6.5–7.0 hours using either halothane or isoflurane with that of an unanaesthetized control group at 2, 4, 6 and 8 days after anaesthesia. They also concluded that maximum deterioration in mental abilities was evident two days afterwards, at which point speed and accuracy scores on a reading test showed marked impairment in both experimental groups. The authors did not report whether the post-intervention tests were given at identical times of day. Their use of a large and complex test battery may also have reduced sensitivity of performance measurements.

Folkard *et al.* (1979) did control for time of day by taking measurements four times a day at four-hourly intervals starting at 08.00 h from herniorrhaphy patients maintained in anaesthesia with either fentanyl or halothane. Their tests of cancellation, addition and reasoning which have been shown to be sensitive, were recorded daily from 2 days before surgery to 6 days afterwards. The absence of a control group complicated analysis but by expressing post-operative performance as a percentage of that on the fifth post-operative day, when presumably practice effects had become minimal, the authors concluded that reasoning abilities remained significantly impaired into the third post-operative day.

A complicated composite performance score derived from a battery of psychological tests was examined before surgery, 4 days and 6 weeks afterwards by Flatt *et al.* (1984). Compared with an unanaesthetized control group tested in their own homes, patients undergoing general anaesthesia displayed impairment which was particularly marked 4 days after surgery.

The suggestion that post-anaesthetic impairment of mental functioning may last for longer than has been generally suspected is borne out by two studies by Herbert *et al.* (1983, 1985). These studies examined the outcome following standard clinical procedures to induce and maintain anaesthesia in male patients undergoing routine, elective surgery for hernia repair. Although such operations are routinely done on a day case basis, the patients for these studies were admitted to hospital wards after surgery to ensure that the testing environment was as standardized as possible.

Patients were asked to complete a four choice serial reaction time test lasting five minutes. The test required the patient to push one of four buttons corresponding geometrically to one of four lights which could be illuminated. Making a response, whether right or wrong, extinguished the light and brought on another in a semi-random sequence (Wilkinson and Houghton, 1975). This test is simple, non-challenging, requires sustained output and maintained concentration and has been shown to be sensitive to anaesthetic agents (Scott *et al.*, 1980). Patients were also asked to complete a series of 18 visual analogue scales to describe their subjective feelings (Herbert *et al.*, 1976).

Both tests were administered on the day before anaesthesia, 90 minutes after regaining consciousness following the operation and at four standard times of day for the first two post-operative days. The tests were given to the patient in bed, with the screens drawn to prevent distraction. In both studies, the reaction time data were compared with the performance of control groups formed from hospitalized, male orthopaedic patients who had not undergone an operation for at least two weeks.

In the first study (Herbert *et al.*, 1983), patients in whom anaesthesia was induced by halothane demonstrated significantly slower reaction times than controls throughout most of the two post-operative days. Patients induced with thiopentone but who breathed spontaneously during anaesthesia also showed impaired reaction times during the second post-operative day. The second study (Herbert *et al.*, 1985) compared performance after induction of anaesthesia using propofol with performance after thiopentone induction. Following thiopentone and compared with controls, performance remained impaired throughout the first post-operative day and during the morning of the second day. Propofol exerted no deleterious effect at any post-operative measurement point (Figure 1).

It seems then, given sufficiently sensitive tests of performance efficiency and given appropriate testing conditions, impairment of mental abilities lasting for at least two post-operative days can be demonstrated after some forms of general anaesthesia. It should be noted that Herbert's studies were based mainly on standard anaesthetic techniques in current use in which patients were given a commonly prescribed premedication dose of diazepam, and induction agents were given in clinically relevant amounts. With maximally sensitive performance measures it becomes possible to assess the influence of other anaesthetic variables such as varying doses of induction

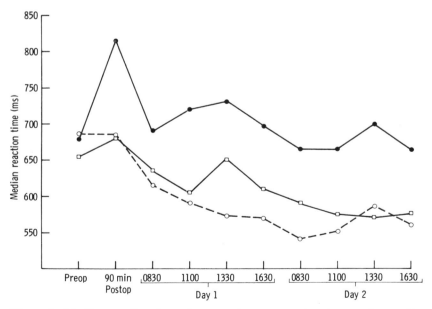

Figure 1. Median reaction times for correct responses at various post-operative points after induction of anaesthesia using propofol (□————□), thiopentone (●————●), and in unanaesthetized controls (○--------○).

agents, premedicants (Cundy and Arunsalam, 1983; Stone *et al.*, 1979) or intra-operative procedures such as hyper- or hypocarbia (Hovorka, 1982). In that way, some of the confusion surrounding the literature on recovery from anaesthesia (Epstein, 1975) might be resolved.

Subjective Estimates of Recovery

An additional question which deserves further investigation is an apparent dissociation between objective and subjective estimates of recovery. Although finding that post-operative performance was maximally impaired on the second post-anaesthetic day, Davison *et al.* (1975) noted strong effects being exerted on scales reflecting depression, fatigue and confusion up to six days post-operatively.

When the dissociation is in that direction, with patients feeling worse than objective tests would predict, the chances of patients resuming potentially hazardous daily activities are probably reduced. It is when patients feel that they are back to normal but objective tests indicate residual impairment that dangerous situations may be more likely to arise.

Egbert *et al.* (1959) were among the early investigators of post-anaesthetic recovery to note that in several instances when subjects judged themselves to be completely recovered, a reaction time test showed that they were not back to normal. The scales used by Herbert *et al.* (1983, 1985) can be differentially weighted to provide measures of self-perceived co-ordination. Conversely, those showing minimal performance effects continued to feel affected by the anaesthetic. This discrepancy is interesting and potentially important since it suggests that patients may not be the best judges of when they are fit enough to resume normal activities.

References

Baskett P and Vickers M (1979) Driving after anaesthetics. *Br. Med. J.*, **1**, 686–7.
Carson IW, Graham J and Dundee JW (1975) Clinical studies of induction agents: XLIII: recovery from althesin—a comparative study with thiopentone and methohexitone. *Br. J. Anaesth.*, **47**, 358–64.
Cundy JM and Arunsalam V (1983) Profile of recovery after general anaesthesia. *Br. Med. J.*, **288**, 2062.
Davison LA, Steinhelber JC, Eger EI and Stevens WC (1975) Psychological effects of halothane and isoflurane anaesthesia. *Anesthesiology*, **43**, 313–24.
Edwards H, Rose EA, Schorow M and King TC (1981) Post-operative deterioration in psychomotor function. *JAMA*, **245**, 1342–3.
Egbert LD, Oech SR and Eckenhoff JE (1959) Comparison of the recovery from methohexital and thiopental anaesthesia in man. *Surg. Gynecol. Obstet.*, **109**, 427–30.
Epstein BS (1975) Recovery from anaesthesia. *Anesthesiology*, **43**, 295–8.
Flatt JR, Birrell PC and Hobbes A (1984) Effects of anaesthesia on some aspects of mental functioning of surgical patients. *Anaesth. Intensive Care*, **12**, 315–24.

Folkard S, Simpson JEP and Glynn CJ (1979) The short- and long-term recovery of mental abilities following minor surgery using different anaesthetic agents. In Oborne DJ, Grunebert MM and Eiser JR (eds). *Research in Psychology and Medicine*, Vol. 2, London: Academic Press.

Gale GD (1976) Recovery from methohexitone, halothane and diazepam. *Br. J. Anaesth.*, **48**, 691–7.

Hannington-Kiff JG (1970) Measurement of recovery from outpatient general anaesthesia with a simple ocular test. *Br. Med. J.*, **3**, 132–5.

Havard JA (1976) Medical aspects of fitness to drive. London: Medical Commission of Accident Prevention.

Herbert M (1978) Assessment of performance in studies of anaesthetic agents. *Br. J. Anaesth.*, **50**, 33–8.

Herbert M, Healy TEJ, Bourke JB, Fletcher IR and Rose JM (1983) Profile of recovery after general anaesthesia. *Br. Med. J.*, **286**, 1539–42.

Herbert M, Johns MW and Dore C (1976) Factor analysis of analogue scales measuring subjective feelings before and after sleep. *Br. J. Med. Psychol.*, **49**, 373–9.

Herbert, M, Makin SW, Bourke JB and Hart EA (1985) Recovery of mental abilities following general anaesthesia induced by propofol ('Diprivan') or thiopentone. *Postgrad. Med. J.*, **61**, (Suppl. 3), 132.

Hindmarch I (1980) Psychomotor function and psychoactive drugs. *Br. J. Clin. Pharmacol.*, **10**, 189–209.

Hockey GRJ and Colquhoun WP (1972) Diurnal variation in human performance: a review. In Colquhoun WP (ed.) *Aspects of Human Efficiency*. London: English Universities Press.

Hovorka J (1982) Carbon dioxide homeostasis and recovery after general anaesthesia. *Acta. Anaesthesiol. Scand.*, **26**, 498–504.

James FM (1969) The effects of cyclopropane anaesthesia without surgical operation on mental functions of normal man. *Anesthesiology*, **30**, 264–72.

Korttila K (1981) Recovery and driving after brief anaesthesia. *Anaesthetist*, **30**, 377–82.

Korttila K, Linnoila M, Ertama P and Hakkinen A (1975) Recovery and simulated driving after intravenous anaesthesia with thiopental, methohexital, proanidid or alphadione. *Anesthesiology*, **43**, 291–9.

Korttila K, Tammisto T, Ertama P, Pfaffli P, Blomgren E and Hakken S (1977) Recovery, psychomotor skills and simulated driving after brief inhalational anesthesia with halothane or enflurane combined with nitrous oxide and oxygen. *Anesthesiology*, **46**, 20–7.

MacKenzie N and Grant IS (1975a) Comparison of the new emulsion formulation of propofol with methohexitone and thiopentone for induction of anaesthesia in day cases. *Br. J. Anaesth.*, **57**, 725–31.

MacKenzie N and Grant IS (1975b) Comparison of propofol with methohexitone in the provision of anaesthesia for surgery under regional blockade. *Br. J. Anaesth.*, **57**, 1167–72.

Nicholson AN (1976) Performance and impaired performance. *Br. J. Clin. Pharmacol.*, **3**, 521–2.

Ogg TW (1972) An assessment of post-operative outpatient cases. *Br. Med. J.*, **4**, 573–6.

Riis J, Lomholt B, Haxholdt O, Kehlet H, Valentin N, Danielsen U and Drybert V (1983) Immediate and long-term recovery from general versus epidural anaesthesia in elderly patients. *Acta Anaesthesiol. Scand.*, **27**, 44–9.

Scott A, Whitnam JG, Wilkinson RT and Whitten JEJ (1980) Assessment of post-operative performance decrement using a serial four-choice reaction-time test. *Br. J. Anaesth.*, **52**, 629–30.

Sikh SS and Dhulia PN (1979) Recovery from general anaesthesia: a simple and comprehensive test for assessment. *Anesth. Analg.*, **58**, 324–6.

Sinclair ME and Cooper GM (1983) Alfentanil and recovery. *Anaesthesia*, **38**, 435–7.

Stone MA, Temperley JM and Marshall EL (1979) The after-effects of intravenous sedation on tasks requiring sustained attention: a study of endoscopy patients over a thirty hour period. In Oborne DJ, Grunebert MM and Eiser JR (eds) *Research in Psychology and Medicine*, Vol. 2, London: Academic Press.

Vickers MD (1965) The measurement of recovery from anaesthesia. *Br. J. Anaesth.*, **37**, 296–302.

Wilkinson RT and Houghton D (1975) Portable four-choice reaction time test with magnetic tape memory. *Behav. Res. Methods Instrumentation*, **7**, 441–6.

Aspects of Recovery from Anaesthesia
Edited by I. Hindmarch, J. G. Jones and E. Moss
© 1987 John Wiley & Sons Ltd

15

Recovery of Cognitive and Psychomotor Function following Anaesthesia. A Review

I. Hindmarch and J. Z. Bhatti

University of Leeds, Leeds

Introduction

A review of the studies that have explored recovery of cognitive and psychomotor function following anaesthesia reveals the existence of a wide variety of putative tests and a range of different methodological procedures (see Appendix). There are many esoteric, though often unvalidated, assessment techniques, as well as a 'common-sense' approach to the measurement of psychological functions to be found in the literature. The diversity and scope of the test and assessment techniques used is evident from a cursory examination of some salient papers. The recall of pre- and post-operative events (Terrall *et al.*, 1969; Brice *et al.*, 1970) would seem to be a parsimonious way of looking at short-term memory and one which has a certain face validity. Similarly, paired associate learning and tests of visual retention have also found favour (Murrin and Nagarajan, 1974; Eckenhoff *et al.*, 1964; Osborne *et al.*, 1967; Riis *et al.*, 1983; Robson *et al.*, 1960; Rollason *et al.*, 1971; Taub and Eisenberg, 1976) and recall of pictures, numbers and verbal materials have all been used to assess changes in memory following anaesthesia (Blundel, 1967; Boas *et al.*, 1983; Grubber and Reed, 1968; Henrie *et al.*, 1961; Ogg *et al.*, 1979; Ogg *et al.*, 1983; Osborne *et al.*, 1967; Parkhouse *et al.*, 1959; Blenkarn *et al.*, 1972). Measures of verbal and intellectual ability have included word learning tests (Eckenhoff *et al.*, 1964; Anderson *et al.*, 1985), reading speed (James, 1969), Wechsler adult intelligence scale (Blundel, 1967; Riis *et al.*, 1983;Robson *et al.*, 1960), Wechsler Belvue stories (Henrie *et al.*, 1961; Parkhouse *et al.*, 1959) and Bennett's clerical test (Eckenhoff *et al.*, 1964).

Motor ability and psychomotor performance have been assessed using a variety of test apparatus. These have included the peg-board (Bahar *et al.*, 1982; Blundel, 1967; Carson, 1975; Denis *et al.*, 1984; Legourneau and Denis, 1983; Machen *et al.*, 1977; Vickers, 1965), the post-box test (Cooper *et al.*, 1983; Craig *et al.*, 1982; Sear *et al.*, 1983; Sinclair and Cooper, 1983; Dixon *et al.*, 1984; Gelfman *et al.*, 1979; Gelfman *et al.*, 1980; Hovorka, 1982; Korttila, 1976; McClure *et al.*, 1983; Newman *et al.*, 1970; White, 1983), and an aiming test (James, 1969). A number of tests has been used to explore the effects of anaesthesia on skills relating to car handling; for example, tracking tests (Denis *et al.*, 1984; Doenicke *et al.*, 1967; Gelfman *et al.*, 1979; Hovorka, 1982; Korttila, 1976; Riis *et al.*, 1983), simulated driving tasks (Green *et al.*, 1963; Egbert *et al.*, 1959; Korttila and Linniola, 1974; Korttila *et al.*, 1975; Wilkinson, 1965) and tracing and maze tests (Anderson *et al.*, 1985; Blundel, 1967; Dixon and Thornton, 1973; Doenicke *et al.*, 1967; Gale, 1974). Sensori-motor co-ordination has been popularly measured using simple reaction time (Azar *et al.*, 1984; Blenkarn *et al.*, 1972; Hovorka *et al.*, 1983; McKercher *et al.*, 1980; Woolman and Orkin, 1968) and choice reaction time (Anderson *et al.*, 1985; Doenicke *et al.*, 1967; Gale, 1974; Grant *et al.*, 1980; Herbert *et al.*, 1983; Korttila, 1976; Male and Johnson, 1984; Scott *et al.*, 1983). The overall efficiency of the CNS as measured by the critical flicker fusion threshold has been also widely employed (Gelfman *et al.*, 1980; Grove *et al.*, 1971; Hovorka, 1982; Hovorka *et al.*, 1983; Korttila and Linniola, 1974; Korttila, 1976; Male and Johnson, 1984; MacKenzie and Grant, 1985a,b; Smith *et al.*, 1967; Vickers, 1965; Azar *et al.*, 1984; James, 1969; Moss *et al.*, 1987; Wernberg *et al.*, 1980). Recovery has also been measured by a coin counting test (Antonios *et al.*, 1984), a static ataxia test (Gale, 1974; Vickers, 1965), letter deletion tasks (Anderson *et al.*, 1985; Antonios *et al.*, 1984; Cooper *et al.*, 1983; Dixon and Thornton, 1973; Edwards *et al.*, 1981; Gelfman *et al.*, 1979, 1980; Riis *et al.*, 1983; Robson *et al.*, 1960; Rollason *et al.*, 1971; Sinclair and Cooper, 1983), and a dichotic listening test (Blenkarn *et al.*, 1972).

The physiological approach to measuring psychological aspects of recovery is reflected in the use of electroencephalograph recordings (Doenicke *et al.*, 1966, 1967); and the Maddox Wing tests (Hannington-Kiff, 1970, 1963).

The diversity of assessment techniques is evident from the above but it must be remembered that in many instances the 'testing procedures' owed more to the enthusiasm of the investigators than to a basic consideration of experimental methodology or the appropriateness of a particular test for a given situation.

Different Classes of Tests

The types of test used to assess recovery from anaesthesia can be arranged into a number of classes. The choice of these classes is not straightforward.

The naive model of behavioural competence described by Michon (1973) provides a convenient breakdown of psychological performance which can be used for test classification. Using this model tests can be described as those that predominantly measure memory, intelligence, psychomotor function and attention, and those that measure physiological characteristics.

Memory

Following anaesthesia, guidance is usually offered to patients on the need to be accompanied, to abstain from alcohol, and not to drive or operate machinery, but this advice is frequently disregarded (Ogg, 1972). The reason for this may well have more to do with the patient being unable to recall the warning rather than a conscious decision to disregard it.

There are three general procedures which have been used to evaluate memory function. Firstly, the questionnaire approach which tests the patient's temporal or spatial orientation and memory for recent events. This is a frequently used technique with patients on neuropsychiatric wards and there are several standardized questionnaires developed for this purpose (Irving *et al.*, 1970). The second method is to obtain ratings of the patient's performance from medical staff working with them (Pattie and Gilleard, 1978). The third and most frequently used method is to devise or adapt cognitive tasks which directly measure rate of acquisition of new information or retention of newly learned material over time. The use of standardized laboratory measures: Wechsler memory scale (Wechsler, 1944) and Kendrick, Parboosingh and Post's synonym learning test (Kendrick *et al.*, 1965) makes comparison of different studies feasible.

Many investigators have made use of paired-associate learning, to assess recognition or recall (Murrin and Nagarajan, 1974; Riis *et al.*, 1983). This test requires the patient to learn, to a given criterion, a series of word pairs which are often associated (e.g. metal–iron). When shown the first member of the pair, patients must be able to state (or recognize from a selection of possible answers) the second member of the pair.

The Benton test of visual retention was used by Eckenhoff *et al.* (1964) and Rollason *et al.* (1971). This test consists of three equivalent sets of 10 cards showing drawings of geometric figures and shapes. The subject is shown a card for 10 seconds and after a delay of 10 seconds is asked to reproduce the design on paper. Scoring is carried out using the number of correct responses out of 10 and the total number of errors.

Other tests of recognition and recall have included free recall of words (Crow and Kelman, 1973), picture recall or recognition (Boas *et al.*, 1983; Blundel, 1967; Grubber and Reed, 1968; Henrie *et al.*, 1961; Ogg *et al.*, 1979, 1983; Osborne *et al.*, 1967; Parkhouse *et al.*, 1959; Riis *et al.*, 1983), story recall (Henrie *et al.*, 1961; Parkhouse *et al.*, 1959), recall of digits of nonsense syllables (Henrie *et al*., 1961; Ghoneim *et al*., 1975; Parkhouse *et al*., 1959) and a vocabulary test (Eckenhoff *et al*., 1964).

These tests have the advantage that they are fairly easy to obtain in standardized forms (e.g. Wechsler Belvue stories could be used as a standardized version of the story recall tests). Unfortunately, this possible advantage that studies could be compared with each other has been made difficult by the wide variety of tests employed. Retention intervals, test materials, distractor tasks and recall test type have not been standardized and often these details are not reported.

Intelligence tests

General intelligence tests are designed for use in a wide variety of situations and are validated against relatively broad criteria. A wide variety of tasks are usually included in the hope of sampling all the important intellectual functions. One commonly used test is the Wechsler adult intelligence scale (Blundel, 1967; Riis *et al*., 1983). Other tests used include Raven's progressive matrices (Blundel, 1967) and the Hunt Minnesota test (Parkhouse *et al*., 1959).

Psychomotor function

Psychomotor tests which are commonly used in assessing recovery from anaesthesia include: the peg-board; post-box; simulated driving; tracking; reaction time and critical flicker fusion.

The first study to use the peg-board to gauge recovery from anaesthesia was conducted by Vickers (1965). The board contained two sets of 48 holes, one set of which was filled with tight fitting pegs. The subject was required to transfer them to the other set of holes as quickly as possible. The score recorded was the number of pegs moved in 45 seconds. Vickers was able to discriminate between two doses of methohexitone (1 mg/kg and 2 mg/kg) in healthy volunteers. The author mentions the problem of practice effects as the subjects had higher scores during the recovery period than they did at pre-test.

In the post-box test patients are required to post as many shapes as possible through the lid of a child's post-box toy within a specified time limit. Craig *et al*. (1982), Sinclair *et al*. (1983), Sear *et al*. (1983) and Cooper *et al*. (1983) carried out studies in which they used the post-box test to measure psychomotor function. In all of these studies comparisons were drawn between different anaesthetic techniques, the only measure of recovery described was the mean time taken for subjects in each group to attain their pre-operative posting score. No information was given as to whether groups were of comparable ability at the pre-test assessment, nor was any allowance made for improvement with practice.

The Trieger dot test requires subjects to connect dots (placed at 12–13 mm intervals) to construct a figure. Scoring involves measuring deviations from a template of the correct figure. The main purpose of this gestalt test is to determine an individual's capacity to experience the act of closure, perceiving a given constellation of stimuli as a whole. The technique has been used to explore retardation, regression, loss of function, organic brain defects and personality deviations. It was also found that fatigue tends to exaggerate disturbances in the gestalt function and that the introduction of CNS depressants leads to sensory motor disturbances which are measurable as the patient recovers from anaesthetic and performance returns to normal. In a study where there were a number of treatment conditions, the Trieger dot test was able to discriminate between them (Newman *et al.*, 1970).

The Lafayette polar pursuit apparatus is one type of tracking task. The patient is required to keep a photoelectric wand inside a moving target for as long as possible. A clock counter connected to the apparatus is inhibited each time the wand leaves the target and the score recorded is the total time required to keep the wand inside the target for 30 seconds (Gelfman *et al.*, 1979; Denis *et al.*, 1984). Tracking tasks have been found to suffer from practice effects complicating interpretation of results.

Other tracking tasks have involved the use of an electric stylus which is used to trace a curving pathway as quickly as possible. The measures taken include deviations from track (time and duration) and the total time required for tracing. Doenicke and his colleagues (1967) concluded that tracking tasks were only useful in detecting gross impairments.

A great variety of simulated driving tasks have been used, some involve tracing around shapes or drawing a pathway out of a maze without coming into contact with any of the edges (Blundel, 1967). The maze test used by Doenicke *et al.* (1967) involved finding the correct path out of a maze as quickly as possible. Dixon and Thornton (1973) made use of a maze test in which the patient was required to trace round a number of adjacent mazes and the number successfully recorded in 60 seconds was noted. Errors were scored when the pencil-drawn solution made contact with the walls of the maze or when it crossed it.

A tracking task used by Gale (1974) comprised a circular turntable which revolved once every 56 seconds and carried a paper disc with a spiral of 240 small circular targets. The targets moved slowly near to the centre and progressively faster towards the periphery. The subject viewed the moving targets through a slit in the lid of the apparatus and was required to draw a pencil line through the spiral line of target shapes. Errors were recorded when targets were missed.

Reaction time tests are popular in the assessment of recovery from anaesthesia because they are easy to learn and quick to administer. Tests can be simple, when a single event is used to signal a single response, or more complex where a choice of responses has to be made according to variable signals. In addition, visual signals, auditory signals or a combination of both have been used to initiate a response.

Wilkinson and Houghton (1975) devised a four-choice reaction time test which has been employed in two studies of recovery from anaesthesia (Herbert *et al.*, 1983; Scott *et al.*, 1983). The apparatus presented subjects with four light emitting diodes organized in a square pattern, one of which was illuminated. Subjects were asked to press a key corresponding geometrically to the illuminated light by using a set of four keys arranged in a similar pattern. By pressing any button, the right or wrong one, the light was extinguished. All responses were recorded on a tape cassette inside the apparatus.

The critical flicker fusion test (CFFT) involves the use of an intermittent light whose flicker rate is increased or decreased within specified limits. As the frequency of flicker increases, a point is reached when it is perceived as continuous, this point being termed the flicker fusion threshold. Conversely when the intermittent light is observed as the frequency of flicker decreases there will be a point when the light that initially appeared constant begins to flicker, the fusion flicker threshold. Most experiments that use this assessment determine the flicker fusion threshold using the method of limits, often taking the mean of three ascending and three descending trials. The test has been shown to give a sensitive measure of central processing of perceptual information (Kleinknecht and Donaldson, 1975) and a good indicator of the sedative action of benzodiazepines (Hindmarch, 1980). In a recent study conducted by Moss *et al.* (1987), CFFT was shown to discriminate between different anaesthetic agents 19 hours after awakening.

The static ataxia test has been used to measure involuntary body sway. A thread is attached to the back of a subject's collar and passed horizontally back through a small ring at one end of a ruled board fixed to the wall. Readings are taken twice for a period of 30 seconds with the subject's feet together and eyes closed (Vickers, 1965).

The visualization test is a pencil and paper test which measures the subject's ability to follow the path of some tangled lines from their point of origin on the left and to label each line with appropriate numbers on the right. The subject's score is taken as the number right in three minutes (James, 1969; Gelfman *et al.*, 1979; and Azar *et al.*, 1984).

Coin counting is a simple test first used by Sikh and Dhulia (1979). In a more recent study a 'float' of 20 coins was prepared containing five each of the coins one, two, five and 10 pence. Seven coins, selected at random, were given to the patient who was required to pick up each coin separately and add up the running total. This procedure was timed, and the average of three attempts was the score recorded for each subject (Antonios *et al.*, 1984).

Tests of attention

Changes in attention levels are measured using tests that involve an individual being presented with a monotonous and uninteresting task. The reduction in attention produced during such a test may be caused by either habituation of physiological responses or by changes in the criteria used by the subject in detecting a signal, or by a combination of these mechanisms (Mackworth, 1970).

The letter deletion task is one measure of attention that is frequently used. In the deletion of p's test the patient is presented with a foolscap sheet containing 58 lines each of 38 closely spaced letters of the alphabet. The task is to delete every letter 'p' on the page, reading from left to right down the page. After three minutes the experimenter counts the number of lines completed and the number of errors (Dixon and Thornton, 1973).

Another test of attention is the dichotic listening task first used by Broadbent (1954) to investigate whether or not subjects could recall anything of material presented to one ear when they were listening to material being presented in the other ear. He gave his subjects three pairs of simultaneous digits, one of each pair to each ear, and then asked them to recall as many digits as they could. Subjects could do this task provided they were allowed to repeat all the digits heard by one ear, followed by those of the other ear. This test was used to measure recovery from anaesthesia by Blenkarn *et al.* (1972).

Physiological measures of recovery

The electroencephalograph (EEG) records the patterns of varying electrical potentials on the scalp due to activity of the cerebral cortex beneath. EEG results have the advantage of not suffering from practice effects, some of the disadvantages include initial cost, scoring results can be time consuming and interpretation of results may not be wholly objective (Ghoneim *et al.*, 1975b). The Maddox Wing measures the balance of the extraocular muscles and gives a sensitive indication of the rate of recovery from general anaesthesia (Hannington-Kiff, 1970). The natural position of rest for the eyes is in divergence with a slight upward displacement and the maintenance of normal vision is an active process, depending largely on the degree of tone in the medial secti muscles. Any reduction in general muscle tone, such as after general anaesthesia, causes divergence of the eyes which can be quantified by using the Maddox Wing. When the patient looks into the instrument his field of vision is divided by oblique and vertical wings such that an arrow is seen by the right eye and a numbered scale by the left. Divergence of the eyes causes the image of the arrow apparently to move along the scale, and the subject is asked to report what number the image of the arrow points to when it has ceased moving. This test has not been used extensively but it appears to be sensitive, reliable and free from practice effects. It does however, rely on patient honesty and co-operation.

Comments

The most difficult and often controversial part of any review involves the summary or the conclusions that are drawn from the information that has been collated. This is particularly the case in the younger scientific disciplines where there are no firmly established paradigms and direct comparisons of work are not easy to conduct. Psychopharmacology, the study of the psychological consequences of pharmacological intervention, is one such discipline.

Research is by its very nature a diverse and progressive activity. Fruitful progression can, however, be hampered when an absence of paradigms make it impossible constructively to compare and contrast different approaches or accurately to evaluate the results from different projects. The literature reviewed reports on experimentation conducted within a clinical setting. This can make good scientific experimentation difficult, but one must accept that more often than not, clinical variables need to take precedence over the control of experimental variables. The present chapter has explored different ways of measuring recovery of psychological function following anaesthesia. The studies reviewed however, are conducted by researchers whose primary interests are in the comparison of anaesthetic agents. For the purposes of the present chapter the type of anaesthetic agent becomes an extra uncontrolled variable. In addition the subject populations, clinical procedures, timing of assessments, types of statistical analyses and a whole host of other variables make direct comparisons of different test systems extremely difficult.

Results

In order to ascertain the value of any given test system in measuring recovery from anaesthesia, an analysis of the more commonly used test procedures has been made. Although the standard of experimentation is rather mixed, all the studies that have had results incorporated in the table were taken from reviewed journals. Brief notes on each of these papers can be found in the Appendix.

Test outcomes have been divided up into three categories; the number of significant discriminations between experimental groups, the number of significant discriminations between baseline/control and experimental groups, and the number of non-significant discriminations. The data obtained is listed in Table 1. Using this data it is possible to calculate an efficiency rating for each test. This is based on the assumption that non-significant discriminations were due to a lack of test sensitivity rather than an actual similarity between the groups tested. The number of successful discriminations (the sum of

Table 1. An analysis of each test results in terms of significant discriminations of experimental groups, significant discriminations between baseline/control and experimental group, and non-significant discriminations

	Total times used	Significant discriminations between experimental groups	Significant discriminations between baseline/control and experimental groups	Non-significant discriminations
Critical flicker fusion threshold	20	11	7	2
Post-box test	16	2	7	7
Letter deletion	13	4	6	3
Picture/object recall and recognition	13	5	5	3
Recall of pre- and post-operative events	12	1	3	8
Peg-board	12	3	1	8
Choice reaction time	12	5	5	2
Simple reaction time	9	3	4	2
Simulated driving tasks	9	6	1	2
Recall of digits/letters/ nonsense syllables	4	1	1	2
WAIS	3	1	1	1
Wechsler Belvue	3	0	2	1
Coin counting	3	3	0	0
Attention tasks	2	1	1	0
EEG	2	2	0	0
Maddox Wing	2	2	0	0

columns 1 and 2) are divided by the total number of times used and multiplied by 100, to give an efficiency rating. It can be argued that an efficiency rating of this type is only a valid measure of a test performance if the test has been used a sufficient number of times, so that evaluations between effectively different groups and under reasonable experimental conditions may be confidently expected. From Table 1 a cut off of at least eight reports appears to provide a suitable confidence limit for test evaluations. Using this criterion six tests appear to be relatively efficient: CFF, choice reaction time, simple reaction time, simulated driving task, letter deletion and picture and object recall/recognition, and three rather less efficient tests; post-box, peg-board and recall of pre- and post-operative events. Although tests like EEG and Maddox Wing appear to be efficient, judgement on their use is being deferred until there have been more reports of their use.

Conclusions

In order for a test to be capable of detecting drug action it needs to be able to measure reliably some aspect of performance that is affected by the drug, and

Table 2. Test efficiency ratings calculated as the percentage of significant discriminating results

	Tests efficiency (%)	No. of times reported
Tests reported less than 8 times		
Critical flicker fusion threshold	90	20
Post-box	56	16
Letter deletion	77	13
Picture/object recall and recognition	77	13
Recall of pre- and postoperative events	33	12
Pegboard	33	12
Choice reaction time	83	12
Simple reaction time	78	9
Simulated driving tasks	78	9
Tests reported less than 8 times		
Recall of digits/letters and nonsense syllables	50	4
WAIS	66	3
Wechsler Belvue	66	3
Coin counting	100	3
Vigilance tasks	100	2
EEG	100	2
Maddox Wing	100	2

to be sensitive enough to pick up small drug-induced changes in performance. The sensitivity and reliability of a test needs to be checked in a laboratory setting prior to use in clinical practice. A third concept that needs to be grasped is that of validity. A test score must be measuring what it is designed to measure. In this case there is a need for tests that can accurately gauge levels of sedation. Again the best method of checking the validity of a test would be to run laboratory studies looking at changes in test performance following different doses of, for example, a sedative–hypnotic.

Sensitivity, reliability and validity are difficult to check and few tests are thoroughly researched. Two exceptions are CFF and choice reaction time which have been shown to detect accurately different levels of sedation (Hindmarch, 1980, 1984). Findings that are reflected in the efficiency rating obtained by these tests.

The test must also be simple enough for it not to have a lengthy training period or for it to suffer from practice effects. In clinical practice there may not be enough time before surgical procedures to train a patient sufficiently to prevent an interaction of practice and anaesthetic effect. In addition any tests used must be easy to set up and run, and the results readily comprehensible without recourse to complex statistics or analyses. Tests used for research purposes may not always be those that are best suited for general use.

The large choice of anaesthetic agents has led to a greatly increased variety of agents, or combination of agents, being administered in outpatient surgery and in dentistry. The pharmacokinetics of each of these agents is studied in great detail prior to their introduction. However, the profiles of recovery shown in psychological tests and pharmacokinetic studies do not always correspond (Ghoneim *et al.*, 1975a). It is, therefore, important that psychological and other performance tests are administered as a safety check to ensure that the effects of anaesthetic agents have been reduced to tolerable levels, before the physician is free from responsibility for his patient. No test, however sensitive to drug effects, can indicate when a patient has recovered, it can only help to isolate those who have failed to recover. The results from these tests can be used as an index of recovery, so that the physician's subjective impression of a patient's cognitive and psychological condition is not the sole basis on which a decision to discharge a patient is taken.

Acknowledgements

The authors wish to express their gratitude to Angie Pain for her help with an earlier manuscript and to Chris Alford for his constructive comments and criticisms.

References

Anderson S, McGuire R and McKeown D (1985) Comparison of the cognitive effects of premedication with hyoscine and atropine. *Br. J. Anaesth.*, **57**, 169–73.

Antonios WRA, Inglis MD and Lees NW (1984) Alfentanil in minor gynaecological surgery; use with etomidate and a comparison with halothane. *Anaesthesia*, **39**, 812–5.

Azar I, Karambelkar DJ and Lear E (1984) Neurologic state and psychomotor function following anaesthesia for ambulatory surgery. *Anesthesiology*, **60**, 347–9.

Bahar B, Dundee JW, O'Neill MP, Briggs LP, Moore J and Merrett JD (1982) Recovery from intravenous anaesthesia—comparison of disoprofol with thiopentone and methohexitone. *Anaesthesia*, **37**, 1171–5.

Blenkarn GD, Briggs G, Bell J and Sugioka K (1972) Cognitive function after hypercapnic hyperventilation. *Anesthesiology*, **37**, 381–6.

Blundel E (1967) A psychological study of the effects of surgery on eighty-six elderly patients. *Br. J. Social Clin. Psychol.*, **6**, 297–303.

Boas RA, Newson AJ and Taylor KM (1983) Comparison of midazolam with thiopentone for outpatient anaesthesia. *NZ Med. J.*, **96**, 210–2.

Brice DD, Hetherington RR and Utting JE (1970) A simple study of awareness and dreaming during anaesthesia. *Br. J. Anaesth.*, **42**, 535–41.

Broadbent DE (1954) The role of auditory localisation in attention and memory span. *J. Exp. Psychol.*, **47**, 191–6.

Carson IW (1975) Recovery from anaesthesia—a review of methods for evaluation of recovery from anaesthesia and a comparative study of the intravenous steriod anaesthetic Althesin (CT 134), with methohexitone and thiopentone. *Proc. R. Soc. Med.*, **68**, 108–10.

Cooper GM, O'Connor M, Mark J and Harvey J (1983) Effects of alfentanil and fentanyl on recovery from brief anaesthesia. *Br. J. Anaesth.*, **55**, 179S.

Craig J, Cooper SM and Sear JW (1982) Recovery from day-case anaesthesia—comparison between methohexitone, Althesin and etomidate. *Br. J. Anaesth.*, **54**, 447–51.

Crow TJ and Kelman GR (1973) Psychological effects of mild acute hypoxia. *Br. J. Anaesth.*, **45**, 335–7.

Cundy JM (1979) Medical aspects of fitness to drive. *Anaesthesia*, **34**, 1056–9.

Denis R, Letourneau JE and Londorf D (1984) Reliability and validity of psychomotor tests as measures of recovery from isoflurane or enflurane anaesthesia in a day-care surgery unit. *Anesth. Analg.*, **63**, 653–6.

Dixon RA and Thornton JA (1973) Tests of recovery from anaesthesia and sedation: Intravenous diazepam in dentistry. *Br. J. Anaesth.*, **45**, 207–15.

Dixon RA, Power SJ, Grundy EM, Lumley J and Morgan M (1984) Sedation for local anaesthesia. Comparison of intravenous midazolam and diazepam. *Anaesthesia*, **39**, 372–6.

Doenicke A, Kugler J, Schellenberger A and Gurtner TL (1966) The use of electroencephalography to measure recovery time after intravenous anaesthesia. *Br. J. Anaesth.*, **38**, 580–90.

Doenicke A, Kugler J and Laub M (1967) Evaluation of recovery and 'street Fitness' by EEG and psychodiagnostic tests after anaesthesia. *Can. Anaesth. Soc. J.*, **14**, 567–83.

Eckenhoff JE, Compton JR, Larson A and Davies RM (1964) Assessment of cerebral effects of deliberate hypotension by psychological measurements. *Lancet*, ii, 711–4.

Edwards H, Rose EA, Schorow M and King TC (1981) Post-operative deterioration in psychomotor function. *JAMA*, **245**, 1342–3.

Egbert LD, Oech SR and Eckenhoff JE (1959) Comparison of the recovery from methohexital and thiopental anaesthesia in man. *Surg. Gynaecol. Obstet.*, **109**, 427–30.

Gale GD (1974) Recovery from methohexitone, halothane and diazepam. *Br. J. Anaesth.*, **48**, 691–8.

Gelfman SS, Gracely RM, Driscoll EJ, Wirdzek PR, Butler DP and Sweet JB (1979) Comparison of recovery tests after intravenous sedation with diazepam–methohexital and diazepam–methohexita and fentanyl. *J. Oral Surg.*, **37**, 391–7.

Gelfman SS, Gracely RM, Driscoll EJ, Butler DP, Sweet JB and Wirdzek PR, (1980) Recovery following intravenous sedation during dental surgery performed under local anaesthesia. *Anesth. Analg.*, **59**, No 10, 775–81.

Ghoneim MM, Mewaldt SP and Ambre J (1975a) Plasma levels of diazepam and mood ratings. *Anesth. Analg.*, **53**, No 2, 173–7.

Ghoneim MM, Mewaldt SP and Thatcher JW (1975b) The effect of diazepam and fentanyl on mental, psychomotor and electroencephalographic functions and their rate of recovery. *Psychopharmacology* (Berlin), **44**, 61–6.

Grant IS, Smith G and Shirley AW (1980) The audiovisual reaction time test. Use in assessment of recovery from Althesin anaesthesia. *Anaesthesia*, **35**, 869–72.

Green R, Long HA and Elliott CJR (1963) A method of studying recovery after anaesthesia—A critical assessment of recovery following methoxitone and thiopentone using a complex performance task. *Anaesthesia*, **18**, 189–200.

Grove-White TG and Kelman GR (1971) Critical flicker frequency after small doses of methohexitone, diazepam and sodium 4-hydroxylbutyrate. *Br. J. Anaesth.*, **43**, 110–2.

Grubber RP and Reed DR (1968) Postoperative anterograde amnesia. *Br. J. Anaesth.*, **40**, 845–9.

Hannington-Kiff JG (1970) Measurement of recovery from outpatient general anaesthesia with a simple ocular test. *Br. Med. J.*, **3**, 132–5.

Hannington-Kiff JGB, Norris W and Nisbet HIA (1963) Objective measurement of sedation III. The reaction timer. *Br. J. Anaesth.*, **35**, 716–9.

Henrie JR, Parkhouse J and Bickford RG (1961) Alteration of human consciousness by nitrous oxide as assessed by electroencephalography and psychological tests. *Anesthesiology*, **22**, 2, 247–59.

Herbert A, Healy TEJ, Bourke JB, Fletcher IR and Rose JM (1983) Profile of recovery after general anaesthesia. *Br. Med. J.*, **286**, 1539–44.

Hindmarch I (1980) Psychomotor function and psychoactive drugs. *Br. J. Clin. Pharmacol.*, **10**, 189–209.

Hindmarch I (1984) Psychometric assessment of the effects of hypnotic drugs. In Priest RG (ed.) *Sleep: An International Mongraph*, 46–55. London: Update.

Hovorka J (1982) Carbon dioxide homeostasis and recovery after general anaesthesia. *Acta. Anaesthesiol. Scand.*, **26**, 498–504.

Hovorka J, Lehtinen AM and Kalli I (1983) Recovery after general anaesthesia for laparoscopy. *Acta. Anaesthesiol. Scand.*, **27**, 396–9.

Irving G, Robinson RA and McAdam W (1970) The validity of zone cognitive tests in the diagnosis of dementia. *Br. J. Psychiatry*, **117**, 149–56.

James FM (1969) The effects of cyclopropane anaesthesia without surgical operation on mental functions of normal man. *Anesthesiology*, **30**, 3, 264–72.

Kleinknect RA and Donaldson D (1975) A review of the effects of diazepam on cognitive and psychomotor performance. *J. Nerv. Ment. Dis.*, **161**, 399–411.

Korttila K (1976) Recovery after intravenous sedation. A comparison of clinical and paper and pencil tests used in assessing late effects of diazepam. *Anaesthesia*, **31**, 724–31.

Korttila K and Linniola M (1974) Skills related to driving after intravenous diazepam, flunitrazepam and droperidol. *Br. J. Anaesth.*, **46**, 961–9.

Korttila K, Linniola M, Ertama P and Hakkinen S (1975) Recovery and simulated driving after intravenous anesthesia with thiopental, methohexita, propanidid or alphadione. *Anesthesiology*, **43**, 291–9.

Legourneau JE and Denis R (1983) The modified GATB(M) as a measure of recovery from general anaesthesia. *Percept. Mot. Skills*, **56**, 451–8.

Machen JB, Ayer WA and Mueller BH (1977) Psychomotor effects of nitrous oxide–oxygen sedation on children. *J. Dent. Child.*, **44**, 51–3.

MacKenzie N and Grant IS (1985a) Comparison of the new emulsion formulation of propofol with methohexitone and thiopentone for induction of anaesthesia in day cases. *Br. J. Anaesth.*, **57**, 725–31.

MacKenzie N and Grant IS (1985b) Comparison of propofol with methohexitone in the provision of anaesthesia for surgery under regional blockade. *Br. J. Anaesth.*, **57**, 1167–72.

Mackworth JF (1970) *Vigilance and Habituation: A Neuropsychological Approach*. Baltimore: Penguin Books.

Male CG and Johnson D (1984) Oral benzodiazepine premedication in minor gynaecological surgery. *Br. J. Anaesth.*, **56**, 499–507.

McClure JH, Brown DT and Wildsmith HAW (1983) Comparison of the iv administration of midazolam and diazepam as sedation during spinal anaesthesia. *Br. J. Anaesth.*, **55**, 1089–92.

McKercher TC, Nelson WJ and Melgaard SA (1980) Recovery and enhancement of reflex reaction time after nitrous oxide analgesia. *J. Am. Dent. Assoc.*, **101**, 785–8.

Michon JA (1973) Human information processing: with and without drugs. *Psychiatria Neurolog.*, **76**, 163–74.

Moss E, Hindmarch I, Pain AJ and Edmonson RS (1987) A comparison of recovery after halothane and altantanil in anaesthesia for minor surgery. *Br. J. Anaesth.*, **59**, 970–7.

Murrin KR and Nagarajan TM (1974) Hyperventilation and psychometric testing. A preliminary study. *Anaesthesia*, **29**, 50–8.

Newman MG, Trieger N, Loskota WJ and Jacobs AW (1970) A comparative study of psychomotor effects of intravenous agents used in dentistry. *Oral Surg.*, **161**, 34–40.

Ogg TW (1972) An assessment of post-operative outpatient cases. *Br. Med. J.*, **4**, 573–6.

Ogg TW, Fischer HBJ, Bethune DW and Collis JM (1979) Day-case anaesthesia and memory. *Anaesthesia*, **34**, 784–9.

Ogg TW, Jennings RA and Morrison CG (1983) Day case anaesthesia for termination of pregnancy. Evaluation of a total intravenous anaesthesia technique. *Anaesthesia*, **38**, 1042–6.

Osborne AG, Bunker JP, Cooper LM *et al.* (1967) Effects of thiopental sedation on learning and memory. *Science*, **157**, 574–6.

Parkhouse J, Henrie JR, Duncan GM and Rome HP (1959) Nitrous oxide analgesia in relation to mental performance. *J. Pharmacol. Exp. Ther.*, **128**, 44–54.

Pattie AH and Gilleard CJ (1978) The two-year predictive validity of the Clifton Assessment Schedule and the Shortened Stockton Geriatric Rating Scale. *Br. J. Psychiatry*, **133**, 457–60.

Riis J, Lomholt B, Haxholdt O *et al.* (1983) Immediate and long-term mental recovery from general versus epidural anaesthesia in elderly patients. *Acta. Anaesthesiol. Scand.*, **27**, 44–9.

Robson JG, Delisle Burns B and Welt PJL (1960) Nitrous oxide memory and time estimation. *Can. Anaesth. Soc. J.*, **7**, No 4.

Rollason WN, Robertson GS, Cordiner CH and Hall DJ (1971) A comparison of mental function in reaction to hypotensive and normotensive anaesthesia in the elderly. *Br. J. Anaesth.*, **43**, 561–5.

Scott WAC, Whitwam JG and Wilkinson RT (1983) Choice reaction time. A method of measuring post-operative psychomotor performance decrements. *Anaesthesia*, **38**, 1162–8.

Sear JW, Cooper GM and Kumar V (1983) The effect of age on recovery. A comparison of the kinetics of thiopentone and Althesin. *Anaesthesia*, **38**, 1158–61.

Sikh SS and Dhulia PN (1979) Recovery from general anaesthesia; a simple and comprehensive test for assessment. *Anesth. Analg.*, **58**, 324–6.

Sinclair ME and Cooper GM (1983) Alfentanil and recovery. *Anaesthesia*, **38**, 435–7.

Smith BL, Allen GD and Perrin EB (1967) A comparison of visual and auditory assessments of recovery from general anaesthesia. *Anesthesiology*, **23**, 596–602.

Taub HA and Eisenberg L (1976) An evaluation of memory under regional anaesthesia with iv lorazepam as a premedicant. *Anesth. Analg.*, **55**, No. 3.

Terrell RD, Sweet WL, Gladfelter JH and Stephen CR (1969) Study of recall during anaesthesia. *Anesth. Analg.*, **48**, 86–90.

Vickers MD (1965) Measurement of recovery from anaesthesia. *Br. J. Anaesth.*, **37**, 296–302.

Wechsler D (1944) *The Measurement of Adult Intelligence* (3rd Edition). Baltimore: Williams & Wilkins.

Wernberg M, Nielsen SF and Hommelgaard P (1980) *Acta. Anaesthesiol. Scand.*, **24**, 86–9.

White PF (1983) Use of continuous infusion versus intermittent bolus administration of fentanyl or ketamine during outpatient anaesthesia. *Anesthesiology*, **59**, 294–300.

Wilkinson BM (1965) Driving ability and reaction times following intravenous anaesthesia. *NZ. Dent. J.*, **61**, 21–6.

Wilkinson RT and Houghton D (1975) Portable four-choice reaction time test with magnetic tape memory. *Behaviour Research Methods and Instrumentation*, **7**, 441–6.

Woolman SB and Orkin LR (1968) Post-operative human reaction time and hypocarbia during anaesthesia. *Br. J. Anaesth.*, **40**, 920–5.

Appendix: Psychological Testing after Anaesthesia

Date	Authors	Number of subjects	Age (years)	Population type	Anaesthetic treatment and dosages	Duration of anaesthesia	Test times	Test results
Recall of pre- and postoperative events								
1963	Feldman	539	15–70	Surgical patients	P.M. either (1) papaveretum + hyoscine (2) pethidine + atropine or (3) promethazine + hyoscine		Questioned following surgery	The papaveretum P.M. was found to be preferred. Pethidine with atropine, especially when given over 60 min before anaesthesia, was the least popular. Promethazine failed to relieve anxiety and hyoscine caused an increased incidence of side-effects.
1969	Terrell et al.	37	22–70 mean = 42	Surgical patients. 14 types of operation	P.M. (short acting barbiturate + atropine or morphine + scopolamine). Ultra-short barbiturate then either (1) halothane (2) methoxyflurane (3) compound 347 (4) cyclopropane (5) ethyl ether or (6) nitrous oxide, oxygen + d-tubocurarine	25–225 min mean = 139 min	Interviewed 2nd and 7th postoperative day	No evidence of recall with either stressful or non-meaningful tape recordings during anaesthesia.

Abbreviations: P.M. = Premedication
P.T. = Pretreatment

Date	Authors	Number of subjects	Age (years)	Population type	Anaesthetic treatment and dosages	Duration of anaesthesia	Test times	Test results
1970	Brice et al.	188	22–77 mean = 48	Surgical patients	Thiopentone (2.5%) either with or without atropine (0.6 mg). Tubo-curarine (30–45 mg), nitrous oxide + oxygen.		2nd and 7th postoperative day	No evidence of recall of piano or choir music. No differences between music + no music groups.
1964	Eckenhoff et al.	36	15–40	Plastic surgery nose/face	P.M. (levorphanol 1–2 mg, promethazine 25 mg, scopolamine 0.4 mg). Thiopentone, suxa-methonium, nitrous oxide + oxygen, halothane + decamethonium. 18 subjects controlled breathing (hypotensive) others spontaneous	88–90 min	P.T. 2–3 days and 6 days	No difference between hypo- and normotensive groups.
1974	Murrin and Nagarajan	16	18–51 mean = 41	Surgical patients 8 types of operations, mainly abdominal.	P.M. (papaveretum + hyoscine, morphine + atropine). suxamethonium, nitrous oxide + oxygen, halothane, muscle relaxant.	Mean = 77 min	P.T. + 2 days	No differences between hyper-ventilated and normal group.
1967	Osborne et al.	24		Paid volunteers	Thiopentone (2.5–3%)		P.T. 30 min	Memory loss for events occurring while under sedation. Memory loss correlated with concentration of thiopentone in venous blood at the time material was learnt.

Year	Author	N	Age	Subjects/Operation	Anaesthesia	Duration	Post-test	Results
1983	Riis et al.	30	60+ mean = 70	Total hip replacement operation	P.M. (pethidine + promethazine) general anaesthesia = thiopentone, nitrous oxide/enflurane + gallamine. Epidural anaesthesia = mepivacaine (2%) and bupivacaine (0.5%) General + epidural = epidural first then general.	Epidural anaesthesia maintained for 24 hrs. General anaesthesia group given pain relief drugs	P.T. 2, 4, 7 days and 3 months	No differences between the three groups at 3–4 days and 3 months following surgery.
1960	Robson et al.	12	27–40	Volunteer subjects	Nitrous oxide (10–approx 40%) and oxygen	10–47 min	While breathing nitrous oxide + oxygen	Subjects were 80% as efficient whilst breathing the gases as they were with air
1971	Rollason et al.	27	Mean = 65	Retropubic hypertrophy patients	P.M. (hyoscine 0.2 mg) sodium thiopentone 2.5%, suxamethonium, nitrous oxide + oxygen, cinchocaine (1:200 solution). Non-hypotensive group given methoxamine		P.T. 5 days, 6 weeks	No differences between normo- and hypotensive groups
1976	Taub and Eisenberg	40	23–65 mean = 40	Surgical procedures (6 different operations)	P.M. (meperidine 50 mg + atropine 0.4 mg and lorazepam 4 mg or placebo). Spinal or epidural anaesthesia	Approx 90 min	24 h later	Stimuli were presented throughout the operation and between the P.M. and surgery. Memory was significantly impaired for all items presented over 20 min after the P.M. was given
1964	Eckenhoff et al.	See earlier	See earlier	See earlier				No significant differences between groups or between pre- and post-test

Date	Authors	Number of subjects	Age (years)	Population type	Anaesthetic treatment and dosages	Duration of anaesthesia	Test times	Test results
1971	Rollason et al.	See earlier	See earlier		See earlier			Scores were ranked. No significant differences
Picture or object recall and recognition								
1967	Blundel	86	70+	Elderly patients undergoing surgery.	Not described		Early test, immediate P.T. then after 1, 2, 3, 4 weeks	Highly significant decrement in performance following surgery
1983	Boas et al.	70	18–70 mean = 49	Surgical patients check cystoscopy	Thiopentone (5 mg/kg) or midazolam (0.125 mg/kg), nitrous oxide + oxygen, halothane	Mean duration 10 min	P.T. 1 h	Midazolam group slightly but not significantly impaired
1968	Grubber and Read	135	10–80 divided into 3 groups 10–40 40–60 60–80	Surgical patients	Two anaesthetic groups and a control. (1) P.M. (atropine 0.4 mg/70 kg, phenobarbitone (100 mg/70 kg) + pethidine (75 mg/70 kg), thiopentone, halothane, nitrous oxide + oxygen. (2) P.M. as above, with amethocaine 1% spinal anaesthetic		P.T. 15 min 60 min + 120 min	Patients undergoing general anaesthesia had significantly greater anaesthesia than spinal patients, when compared with control
1961	Henrie et al.	18	18–50 mean = 30.5	Volunteer subjects	Nitrous oxide + oxygen	Mean = 30 min	P.T. 10 min (from start of administration) + 30 min after administration	Marked impairment between performance of the group when breathing gas and when breathing air

Year	Author	N	Age	Type	Anaesthetic		Timing	Results
1979	Ogg et al.	52	Mean = 23	Day case surgical patients	Either fentanyl, methohexitone nitrous oxide + oxygen or methohexitone, nitrous oxide and oxygen with trichlorethylene if necessary. (Control group no operation)	Group 1 = 10.9 min. Group 2 = 10.0 min	P.T. 1 h + 3 h	Both anaesthetic groups were impaired when compared to the control group at 1 h. By 3 h both recovered
1983	Ogg et al.	50	16–40	Termination of pregnancy operations	Fentanyl (1.5 g/kg) + methohexitone (1%) + lignocaine (1%) with either nitrous oxide + oxygen + trichloroethylene or methohexitone (0.25 mg/kg) + oxygen (healthy nurses and in-patients used for control)	Trichloroethylene group Mean = 8.7 min Fentanyl group Mean = 8.1 min	P.T. 1 h, 2 h	Both anaesthetic groups showed significant depression of memory recall at 1 h (according to text, but not in results table)
1967	Osborne et al.	See earlier			See earlier			Amnesia was greatest for material learnt under highest levels of sedation. Amnesic effect of thiopentone not retroactive
1960	Parkhouse et al.	24	18–50	Volunteer subjects	Nitrous oxide (20%, 30% or 40%) and oxygen	10 min	Immediate + 30 min	Only slightly slower learning with 20% nitrous oxide, slightly more deterioration following 30% and maximal impairment after 40%

Date	Authors	Number of subjects	Age (years)	Population type	Anaesthetic treatment and dosages	Duration of anaesthesia	Test times	Test results
1972	Blenkarn et al.	6	22–31	Volunteer subjects	Thiopentone, nitrous oxide d-tubocurarine	125 min or less	P.T. 90 min after anaesthesia then daily for 4 days	Anaesthesia with hypocapnia produced no more impairment than anaesthesia alone. 90 min after treatment, performance in this test not affected
1961	Henrie et al.	See earlier	See earlier		See earlier			When breathing gas performance impaired
1975(a) Ghoneim et al.		10	21–25 Mean = 22	Volunteer subjects	Diazepam (10 or 20 mg) or fentanyl (0.1 or 0.2 mg) or placebo		P.T. 2 h, 6 h, 8 h	No significant drug effect or interactions

Recall of digits, letters or nonsense syllables

Date	Authors	Number of subjects	Age (years)	Population type	Anaesthetic treatment and dosages	Duration of anaesthesia	Test times	Test results
1960	Parkhouse et al.	See earlier	See earlier		See earlier			Worst performance following 40% nitrous oxide, impairment still present with 30% and only slight following 20%
1964	Eckenhoff et al.	See earlier	See earlier		See earlier			No differences between hypotensive and normotensive groups

132

Year	Author		Age	Subjects	Anaesthetic/drug	Test timing	Results
1985	Anderson et al.	30	22–55	Dilatation and curettage patients	P.M. (either hyoscine 0.4 mg or atropine 0.6 mg or placebo). Thiopentone 500 mg, nitrous oxide, oxygen + halothane	P.T. 30 min after P.M. then 1 h and 3 h after return to the ward	Delayed recall of word lists presented after drug administration was impaired in the group who received halothane. This group was also worse (but not significantly) at immediate recall in tests 2 and 3
1969	James	18	21–24	Healthy volunteers	Cyclopropane anaesthesia (5–40%)		No significant differences between the results after receiving cyclopropane and the P.T.

Intelligence tests
Wechsler Adult Intelligence Scale

Year	Author			Subjects	Anaesthetic/drug		Results
1967	Blundel	See earlier			See earlier		(Arithmetic, similarities, vocabulary, block design subtests). The arithmetic and block design subtests both showed significant impairment in the surgical group when compared with the control group

133

Date	Authors	Number of subjects	Age (years)	Population type	Anaesthetic treatment and dosages	Duration of anaesthesia	Test times	Test results
1983	Riis *et al.*	See earlier			See earlier			(Block design sub-test.) Scores showed no significant differences between general anaesthesia, epidural anaesthesia and the control group both before and after surgery
1960	Robson *et al.*	See earlier			See earlier		See earlier	Digit span, mental arithmetic, block design, digit symbol subtests used. Following nitrous oxide these tests were performed with 69%, 50%, 57% and 62% of normal efficiency respectively
Wechsler Belvue stories								
1961	Henrie *et al.*	See earlier			See earlier			Scores from the immediate and delayed testing of recognition showed that registration and recall of the stories were significantly impaired. Forgetting was also more rapid following gas

Year	Author	n	Mean age	Patients	Method	Mean	Test	Results
1960	Parkhouse et al.	See earlier	See earlier	See earlier			See earlier	Immediate and delayed recall scores showed no significant differences between compressed air and 20% nitrous oxide. Following 30% and 40% nitrous oxide, impairment was significantly greater than following compressed air
1964	Eckenhoff et al.	See earlier	See earlier	See earlier			See earlier	No significant differences between hypotensive and normotensive groups
Tests of motor skill **Peg-board**								
1982	Bahar et al.	50	Mean = 32	Minor gynaecological surgical patients	Induction using either propofol (2 or 3 mg/kg) thiopentone (4 or 6 mg/kg) or methohexitone (1.5 mg/kg)	Mean = 4 min	P.T. then tested until pegboard score returned to P.T. value	No significant differences between the five groups
1967	Blundel	See earlier		See earlier				Male patients significantly impaired. No significant differences between surgical and and control groups
1975	Carson			Patients for short surgical procedures	Althesin or methohexitone or thiopentone		P.T. then pegboard score returned to P.T. value	Althesin group tested until required significantly longer to reach their P.T. performance

Date	Authors	Number of subjects	Age (years)	Population type	Anaesthetic treatment and dosages	Duration of anaesthesia	Test times	Test results
1984	Denis et al.	30	20–68 mean = 36	Patients undergoing minor surgery (control group of nurses)	P.M. (meperidine 1 mg/kg + atropine sulphate 0.4 mg). Thiopentone, succinylcholine with either nitrous oxide, oxygen and isoflurane or nitrous oxide, oxygen and enflurane	25–150 min, mean = 50 min	P.T. 90, 150 and 210 min	Control group showed a significant improvement. Baseline scores of control and experimental group differed. By test four the experimental group had not reached their P.T. performance
1983	Legourneau and Denis	23	16–59 mean = 32	Patients undergoing general anaesthesia and surgery. (Control group of relatives and students n = 23.)	P.M. (meperidine, in 6 patients) Infusion with either pentothal or fentanyl or a combination of both. Maintenance with either nitrous oxide, oxygen and enflurane, or halothane. Some patients received d-tubocurarine, succinylcholine or atropine	25–120 min mean = 52 min	P.T. 90, 150 and 210 min	Results of the control group were significantly different over the four tests. The experimental groups were significantly impaired when compared with the control, at all test times
1977	Machen et al.	56	2 groups 4–8 9–13	Patients undergoing restorative dental treatment	Experimental group received a local anaesthetic and nitrous oxide and oxygen. (Control group received local anaesthetic)	All less than 40 min	P.T. immediately and 20 min after treatment	No significant differences between any of the groups

136

1965	Vickers	8	Volunteer subjects	Either thiopentone 2.5 mg/kg or 5.0 mg/kg or methohexitone 1 mg/kg or 2 mg/kg		P.T. then every 15 min until P.T. values obtained	No tests of significance were carried out. A practice effect was noted. Recovery times were 30–60 min after methohexitone (1 mg/kg) and 45–90 min after methohexitone (2 mg/kg). After thiopentone (2.5 mg/kg) recovery took 45–90 min and after thiopentone (5 mg/kg) 135–210 min
1983	Cooper et al.	100	18–50 mean = 32	Patients undergoing dilatation to the uterine cervix	Induction with methohexitone (1.5 mg/kg) + either (1) no analgesic (2) fentanyl (1.5 μg/kg) (3) alfentanil (8 μg/kg) (4) alfentanil (12 μg/kg) (5) alfentanil (16 μg/kg)	Mean = 7.8 min	P.T. then tested every 5 min after waking up until P.T. score attained	No significant differences between the groups
1982	Craig et al.	100	16–50 mean = 32	Patients undergoing dilatation to the cervix	Either methohexitone (1.5 mg/kg) with 10 mg increments when required or Althesin (0.6 mg/kg), with increments of Althesin when required. Half of each group was also given fentanyl (100 μg) before their induction dose. The fifth group received etomidate (0.3 mg/kg) with fentanyl (100 μg)	Mean = 8.8 min	P.T. then tested every 5 min after waking up until P.T. score attained	Times to complete the post-box test were significantly longer in the etomidate group than following methohexitone or Althesin alone. No other significant differences

Date	Authors	Number of subjects	Age (years)	Population type	Anaesthetic treatment and dosages	Duration of anaesthesia	Test times	Test results
1983	Sear et al.	80	18–85 Young group mean = 36 yrs Old group mean = 58 yrs	Patients undergoing dilatation and curettage	Either thiopentone (4 mg/kg) or Althesin (0.6 mg/kg). Maintenance was with (67%) nitrous oxide in oxygen + (1.5%) halothane	Mean = 8.1 min	P.T. then tested every 5 min after waking up until P.T. score attained	No significant differences between scores of both Althesin groups and the young thiopentone group. The older thiopentone group required significantly longer to reach the P.T. scores
1983	Sinclair and Cooper	40	18–50	Patients undergoing dilatation to the uterine cervix	Either Althesin (50 μg/kg) with increments of 0.5 ml and alfentanil (8 μg/kg); or methohexitone (1.5 mg/kg) with increments of 10 mg and alfentanil (8 μg/kg)	Mean = 9.8 min	P.T. then tested every 5 min after waking up until P.T. score attained	No significant differences between the two groups
1984	Dixon et al.	100	Mean = 53	Patients undergoing local (regional block) anaesthesia	Either diazepam (0.5 mg/kg) or midazolam (0.08 mg/kg), with local anaesthetic		P.T. then 4 h, 6 h, and 24 h following anaesthesia	No significant differences between the two drugs

138

Post-box test

	n	Age	Subjects	Drug/dose	Duration	Test times	Results
1979 Gelfman *et al.*	207 (62 patients did experiment twice)	Mean = 23	Patients requiring surgery on their molar teeth (control group received only local anaesthetic)	Either diazepam (15 mg) and methohexitone (30–40 mg), or fentanyl (0.04–0.05 mg) diazepam (12.5 mg) and methohexitone (40 mg), given with local anaesthetic	20–30 min	P.T. after anaesthetic and before surgery, immediately after surgery, 3 h and 1 week later	Immediately after surgery both experimental groups were significantly more impaired than the control. There was no significant difference between the two experimental groups at this or other test times
1980 Gelfman *et al.*	94 (all subjects did experiment twice, once in each condition) (control group n = 40 had only local anaesthetic	18–35 mean = 24	Patients undergoing molar extractions	Either diazepam (15 mg) and methohexitone (20–200 mg) or diazepam (12.5 mg) methohexitone (20–200 mg) and fentanyl (0.1 mg), given with local anaesthetic		P.T. after anaesthetic and before surgery, immediately after surgery, 3 h and 1 week later	Statistically significant decrements in performance immediately and 1 h postoperatively for both drug combinations. No difference between two experimental groups

Date	Authors	Number of subjects	Age (years)	Population type	Anaesthetic treatment and dosages	Duration of anaesthesia	Test times	Test results
1982	Hovorka	60	Group 1 aged over 60 Mean = 66 Group 2 aged under 46 Mean = 40	Patients undergoing abdominal gynaecological surgery	P.M. atropine (0.01 mg/kg) and pethidine (1 mg/kg). Thiopentone (3.4–4.2 mg/kg) nitrous oxide and oxygen and increments of fentanyl (0.05–0.1 mg)		P.T. 1 h, 2 h, 3 h, and 24 h postoperatively	No significant differences between the age groups in any of the conditions
1976	Korttila	12	Mean age = 22	Volunteer students	Diazepam (0.15 mg/kg)		P.T. 30 min and 150 min after injection	No significant impairment when compared with P.T. at both test times
1983	McClure et al.	20	Mean age = 44	Patients undergoing spinal anaesthesia	P.M. temazepam (10 mg). Either midazolam (0.1 mg/kg) or diazepam (0.2 mg/kg), with increments of each when required. All patients received 0.5% plain bupivacaine (4 ml)	Mean = 57 min	P.T. 2 h and 3 h	Both groups showed marked impairment at the 2 h test but were improved by 3 h. No significant differences between the groups
1970	Newman et al.	57		Patients undergoing oral surgery	Either phenobarbitone or hydroxyzine and meperidine with scopolamine or atropine and/or methohexitone. All patients received local anaesthesia		P.T. immediately after coming round and 10 min later. A final test was done when patient considered fit for discharge	Results showed when compared to P.T. each successive test produced less errors

140

1983	White	100	Mean ages for the groups = 22–25	Patients for gynae-cological surgery	P.M. droperidol (0.5 mg) and glycopyrrolate (0.2 mg). Thiopentone (4 mg/kg) with either fentanyl (50 μg bolus or 2 μg/ml given by infusion at a rate of 0.1 μg/kg/min) or ketamine (25 mg bolus or 1 mg/ml given by infusion at a rate of 50 μg/kg/min). All patients nitrous oxide in oxygen	Mean = 27 min	P.T. 30, 60, 90, and 120 min	More rapid recovery following infusion in both drug groups. Ketamine infusion group was signifi-cantly better than the bolus for 90 min after treatment, and in the fentanyl group the infusion patients were significantly better for 60 min. Generally, ketamine scores were slower than the fentanyl scores
1969	James	See earlier	See earlier		See earlier			No significant differ-ences between P.T. and scores following cyclopropane
1984	Denis et al.	See earlier	See earlier		See earlier			Both the control and experimental groups showed significant improvement over the four trials. The experimental group did show significant impairment when compared to the control group

Date	Authors	Number of subjects	Age (years)	Population type	Anaesthetic treatment and dosages	Duration of anaesthesia	Test times	Test results
1967	Doenicke et al.	81		Healthy volunteer subjects	Either (1) thiopentone (3.5–7 mg/kg) alone or with halothane; (2) thio-butabarbitone (3.5–7 mg/kg); (3) methohexitone (2 mg/kg); (4) propanidid (7 mg/kg) with (i) halo-thane, (ii) nitrous oxide and oxygen, (iii) ether and oxygen, (iv) nitrous oxide and halothane, (v) alone, (6) CI 581 (2 mg/kg). In some cases alcohol was also used		P.T. 90 and 150 min	No statistically signi-ficant differences between groups. The tracking test was only found to be useful in detecting gross impairments
1979	Gelfman et al.	See earlier	See earlier		See earlier			Despite practice effects the results showed significant deficits in the two experimental groups up to 3 h after surgery
1982	Hovorka	See earlier	See earlier		See earlier			The time to complete the tracking test proved to be more sensitive than the error measure. The older age group was found to be signifi-cantly impaired in all three conditions at the 1, 2 and 3 h times of testing

142

Year	Author		Subjects	Age	Subject type	Drug/dose	Recovery	Testing	Results
1976	Korttila	See earlier							There was a significant increase in the error rate of the experimental group 150 min after diazepam when compared to P.T.
1983	Riis et al.	See earlier							The test was not analysed individually, but as part of an attention score. All three groups showed a significant decrement in performance 2 days after surgery, but there were no significant differences between the groups
1963	Green et al.		20	20–25	Student volunteers (all subjects received both treatments)	Methohexitone (0.88 mg/kg) or thiopentone (2.64 mg/kg)	Mean = 2 min 11 sec	P.T. then 10, 20, 30, 40 and 70 min after injection	No significant differences on any of the measures
1959	Egbert et al.		14		Healthy volunteers (each subject studied four times)	Methohexitone (200–300 mg) thiopentone (70–110 mg)	Mean = 17 min 42 sec	P.T., tested until performance returned to normal	Subjects who received methohexitone recovered significantly faster

143

Date	Authors	Number of subjects	Age (years)	Population type	Anaesthetic treatment and dosages	Duration of anaesthesia	Test times	Test results
Simulated driving tasks								
1974	Korttila and Linnoila	62	Mean age = 22	Healthy student volunteers	(1) diazepam (0.3 mg/kg), (2) diazepam (1.5 mg/kg) and pethidine (1 mg/kg) (3) flunitrazepam (0.03 mg/kg) (4) flunitrazepam (0.015 mg/kg) and pethidine (1 mg/kg), (5) droperidol (5 mg), (6) droperidol (5 mg) and fentanyl (0.2 mg)	Mean = 45 min	P.T. tested 4 h, 6 h, 8 h and 10 h	In the first tracking test (fixed speed), mistakes in co-ordination were significantly increased for up to 10 h after droperidol and flunitrazepam and 6 h after diazepam. Second test showed that both droperidol conditions significantly increased the number of mistakes at all times
1975	Korttila et al.	50	Mean age = 22	Healthy volunteers	2.5% thiopentone (6.0 mg/kg) or 1% methohexitone (2.0 mg/kg) or 5% propanidid (6.6 mg/kg) or Althesin (85 μg/kg) (control group received nothing)	Mean = 6 min	P.T. 2 h, 4 h, 6 h and 8 h	Clinical recovery was faster after propanidid and methohexitone than the other two agents. Driving performances remained significantly impaired for 6 h after methohexitone and reaction times 8 h after thiopentone were significantly worse than in control group. Propanidid produced no impairment in any tests

144

Year	Author	Number	Age	Subjects	Drug/dose	Timing	Results
1965	Wilkinson	10	17–41 mean = 24	Volunteer subjects	2% methohexitone (5–8.5 cm^3)	P.T. 5 min, 10 min, and 20–25 min following injection	By the final test, subjects were attaining faster times than at P.T. No tests of significance were carried out, but impairment was observed in the first test.
1985	Anderston et al.	See earlier	See earlier	See earlier	See earlier		Hyoscine group were significantly slower than patients who received no P.M. at the 1 h test. By the 3 h test the hyoscine group were significantly slower that the atropine group. There were no significant differences between the error scores of each group.
1967	Blundel	See earlier	See earlier	See earlier	See earlier		No differences in pre- and post-operative performance of surgical group. The old people in a home did, however, show a deterioration after their admission.
1973	Dixon and Thornton	148		Dental patients	Diazepam (0.12–0.32 mg/kg) and local analgesia or local analgesia alone	Earlier visit, immediate P.T. immediately after surgery and 1 week later	Diazepam patients were significantly impaired compared with their P.T. The control group had significantly improved the number of mazes completed without increasing their error rate

Date	Authors	Number of subjects	Age (years)	Population type	Anaesthetic treatment and dosages	Duration of anaesthesia	Test times	Test results
1967	Doenicke *et al.*	See earlier	See earlier		See earlier			150 min after receiving the anaesthetic agents, the propanidid and alcohol group were significantly less impaired than the methohexitone and alcohol group
1976	Gale	52	14–59 Mean age = 30	Patients for short dental procedures	(1) Methohexitone (1.07–1.79 mg/kg) (2) halothane, nitrous oxide and oxygen (3) as above, but for longer. (4) diazepam (0.28–5.1 mg/kg) and local analgesia (5) no anaesthetic	Mean duration for (1) 4.6 min, (2) 6.2 min, (3) 32 min, and (4) 47 min	P.T. then 15–20 min, 20–25 min, 50–75 min, 2 h, 3 h, and 24 h after initial recovery	Practice effect obvious in control group. On slow tracking, the short halothane, and methohexitone groups had improved on their P.T. scores by 25 min test. On rapid tracking all groups demonstrated impairment and in the long halothane group this lasted over an hour
1984	Azar *et al.*	120	Mean age = 34	Patients undergoing short procedures, mainly dilatation and curettage	P.M. diazepam (0.08 mg/kg) all patients received thiopentone (4 mg/kg) and nitrous oxide and oxygen with either (1) fentanyl (2 μg/kg) or (2) enflurane (3.4%) or (3) isoflurane (2.6%)	Mean duration = 14 min	P.T. 1 h and 2 h	At the 1 h test all three groups were impaired when compared to P.T. at the 1 h test. By 2 h only the enflurane group displayed a significant degree of impairment

146

Study	Number	Subjects		Timing of test	Results
Simple reaction time 1972 Blenkarn et al.	See earlier	See earlier			No significant difference between the two experimental groups, both were significantly impaired at the 90 min test
1981 Edwards et al.	40	Patients undergoing routine elective operations (control group on bed-rest or nurse volunteers)	Not described	P.T. then post-operative days 2–10	A significant increase in reaction times was noted for 7 days following surgery
1975(b) Ghoneim et al.	See earlier	See earlier			Median reaction time score showed no differences between the groups, but analysis of the standard deviations showed that diazepam increased response variability significantly more than fentanyl in the simple task, and more than all conditions in the choice reaction time task

147

Date	Authors	Number of subjects	Age (years)	Population type	Anaesthetic treatment and dosages	Duration of anaesthesia	Test times	Test results
1963	Hendry et al.	113		Patients undergoing minor gynae-cological procedures	Not described (four standard drugs given for P.M.)		Before and after sedation	Only when sedation was rated to be 'good' did the reaction time results correlate well with observations of sedation
1982	Hovorka	See earlier	See earlier		See earlier			No significant post-operative differences between any of the conditions
1983	Hovorka et al.	30	Mean age = 30 yrs	Patients undergoing gynae-cological laparoscopy	P.M. pethedine (1mg/kg) + atropine (0.1 mg/kg). Either thiopentone (4.5 mg/kg), fentanyl (0.002 mg/kg) or enflurane. Both groups received nitrous oxide and oxygen + succinylcholine	Mean = 45 min	P.T., 1 h, 2 h and 3 h post-operatively	The fentanyl group were significantly impaired when com-pared with the en-flurane group at both the 1 and 2 h tests. By the final test only the enflurane patients had attained their P.T. performance
1980	McKercher et al.	15		Student volunteers	Nitrous oxide + oxygen for 15 min then 100% oxygen for 5 min		P.T. then 5, 10, 20, and 30 min	While breathing nitrous oxide reaction times were significantly longer than those of P.T. and by the last test they were signifi-cantly faster

| 1968 | Woolman and Orkin | 37 | Patients undergoing short surgical procedures | Half hypocarbic and half normocarbic | P.T. then between 3 and 6 days following surgery | The hypocarbic group demonstrated impaired performance for 3–6 days following surgery, both compared to P.T. and the normocarbic group |
| 1985 | Anderson *et al.* | See earlier | See earlier | See earlier | | In the 3 h test, the hyoscine patients were significantly slower than those in the placebo and atropine groups in their total choice reaction time scores |

Choice reaction time

| 1967 | Doenicke *et al.* | See earlier | See earlier | See earlier | | No significant differences were observed between groups when assessed with this test |
| 1976 | Gale | See earlier | See earlier | See earlier | | Auditory reaction times were significantly impaired after methohexitone at the 50–75 min test and 1 h after diazepam. Visual reaction time results showed no significant changes for any of the groups |

Date	Authors	Number of subjects	Age (years)	Population type	Anaesthetic treatment and dosages	Duration of anaesthesia	Test times	Test results
1980	Grant *et al.*	58 (29 patients used as a control)	26–58 years	Patients undergoing minor surgical procedures (dilatation and curettage)	Althesin (2.5–4 ml), nitrous oxide, oxygen + halothane (0.5–1.0%)	8–15 min Mean = 10.9 min	P.T., 40 min, 100 min + 160 min after induction	No significant differences between the test times in the control group. At the 40 min test, the experimental group were significantly impaired compared with the control group and their P.T. score
1985	Grant *et al.*	80		Patients undergoing orthopaedic surgery	Propofol, methohexitone and thiopentone using three different techniques		30, 60, 90, 120 and 240 min	Rapid recovery following propofol
1983	Herbert *et al.*	55	Mean age = 49	Patients undergoing hernia repair operation	P.M. diazepam 10 mg. Thiopentone (250 mg), halothane (0.5–1.5%), nitrous oxide + oxygen). Some patients were given suxamethonium + alcuronium and were intubated to control their breathing. Others received halothane to induce anaesthesia, and breathed spontaneously. The third group breathed spontaneously and did not receive halothane		P.T. 90 min after regaining consciousness + tests on the 1st + 2nd postoperative days at 8.30, 11.00, 13.30 + 16.30 h	The experimental groups showed a gradual return to pre-surgical response levels over the 2 days. The groups who received halothane and those who breathed spontaneously were still impaired at all test times on day 2 when compared with the control group

150

Year	Author	N	Age	Treatment	Route	Measurement times	Results
1976	Korttila	See earlier	See earlier	See earlier			A significant increase in total reaction times was observed 150 min following diazepam, when compared with P.T.
1985(a)	MacKenzie et al.	60	18–65	Propofol 2.5 mg/kg, 1% methohexitone 1.5 mg/kg, 2.5% thiopentone 5 mg/kg	iv over 20 sec	Baseline, 30, 60, 90 and 120 min	All treatments caused significant impairment at 30 min. Thiopentone caused impairment for 90 min
1985(b)	MacKenzie et al.	40	16–65	Propofol 2.5 mg/kg, methohexitone 1.5 mg/kg	iv	30, 60, 90, 120 and 240 min	Impairment found following both treatments at 30 and 60 min
1984	Male and Johnson	150	17–69 mean = 41 years	P.M. (1) diazepam 10 mg, (2) oxazepam 30 mg (3) lorazepam 2 mg (4) clobazam 20 mg (5) placebo. 2.5% thiopentone (200–350 mg), nitrous oxide + halothane (up to 2.5%) in oxygen	5–15 min	P.T., 1 h after P.M., 2 h, 4 h and 16–24 h after operation	The group who received lorazepam were found to be significantly slower at the 2 h test in both total and recognition reaction times. No other treatments produced a significant decrement
1987	Moss et al.	44		Patients undergoing minor gynaecological surgery	Halothane or alfentanil		Full recovery at 19 h post op. with alfentanil. Continued sedation with halothane at same time

151

Date	Authors	Number of subjects	Age (years)	Population type	Anaesthetic treatment and dosages	Duration of anaesthesia	Test times	Test results
1983	Scott et al.	39	Mean age = 32.7	Patients undergoing minor gynae-cological procedures, control group of hospitalized patients not being operated on	Either (1) thiopentone (4.5 mg/kg), nitrous oxide + halothane or (2) fentanyl, methohexitone (3.2 mg/kg), nitrous oxide, oxygen + incre-mental doses of metho-hexitone. (Atropine + ergometrine were used at times)	Group (1) mean = 15.5 min Group (2) mean = 14.9 min	P.T., 2 h, 4 h, 6 h, 8 h + 24 h following surgery	Control subjects showed a significant improvement with practice. Both experi-mental conditions showed significant impairment for the first 4 h. Thiopentone subjects appeared recovered at the 6 h test but were signifi-cantly impaired at the 8 h test. After 24 h there were no significant differ-ences between the control and experi-mental groups
CRT 1980	Wernberg et al.	6 male 4 female	See earlier	Healthy volunteers	0%, 10%, 20% and 30% nitrous oxide	15 min		No significant results
The critical flicker fusion (CFF) test 1979	Gelfman et al.	See earlier		See earlier				Experimental groups both showed signifi-cantly decreased scores immediately and 3 h after surgery. No significant differ-ences between the two experimental groups

152

Year	Author	Agent/dose	N	Age	Subjects	Results
1980	Gelfman et al.	See earlier	See earlier			No significant changes in placebo group. The two experimental groups both had significantly decreased scores immediately + 3 h post-operatively, but did not differ from each other
1985	Grant et al.	See earlier	See earlier			No effects with propofol. Methohexitone induced impairment for 30 min, thiopentone induced effects for 90 min. In the intermittent bolus study propofol effects were found at all test times, methohexitone effects for 120 min
1971	Grove-White and Kelman	Either (1) methohexitone (0.15 mg/kg) (2) diazepam (0.05 mg/kg) + (3) sodium 4-hydroxybutyrate (10 mg/kg)	10	19–22	Volunteer subjects	P.T. 5 min, 15 min, 30 min and 90 min after injection. Significant reduction in CFF scores following all three agents. Recovery was fastest in the sodium 4-hydroxybutyrate group (30 min) and took up to 90 min in the diazepam and methohexitone groups

Date	Authors	Number of subjects	Age (years)	Population type	Anaesthetic treatment and dosages	Duration of anaesthesia	Test times	Test results
1982	Hovorka	See earlier			See earlier			There were no significant differences between the two age groups, but the hypocarbic sub-group were consistently more impaired than the other two sub-groups, and the normocarbic more impaired than the hypercarbic group, throughout the testing period
1983	Hovorka et al.	See earlier			See earlier			The fentanyl group were significantly more impaired after surgery than the en-flurane group. Both groups were impaired when compared with their P.T. scores, but had recovered by the 3 h test
CFF 1981	Korttila et al. Study 1	22	Mean age = 23	Healthy volunteers	30% nitrous oxide	2 periods of 40 min separated by 45 min	2, 12, 22 and 32 min after administration	CFF failed to show drug effects
	Study 2	8		Healthy volunteers	30% nitrous oxide and oxygen in cross-over design	As for study 1	As for study 1	

154

1974	Korttila and Linnoila	See earlier	See earlier	After every treatment, scores were significantly decreased for up to 6 h, but following droperidol impairment was still obvious 10 h after treatment
1976	Korttila	See earlier	See earlier	No significant changes were observed in the CFF scores following diazepam
1985(a)	MacKenzie et al.	See earlier		No impairment with propofol, impairment with methohexitone lasted for 30 min and with thiopentone for 90 min
1985(b)	MacKenzie et al.	See earlier		CFF threshold reduced following propofol at all test times, with methohexitone impairment for 2 h
1984	Male and Johnson	See earlier	See earlier	Lorazepam was found to produce a significant reduction in CFF scores immediately after premedication and at all the postoperative tests. None of the other premedications produced any impairment

155

Date	Authors	Number of subjects	Age (years)	Population type	Anaesthetic treatment and dosages	Duration of anaesthesia	Test times	Test results
1987	Moss *et al.*	See earlier						Drop in CFF immediately following both treatments. Halothane group were still impaired 19 h after operation
1967	Smith *et al.*	40	Mean age = 28	Patients undergoing minor gynaecological or oral surgery	Either (1) halothane + oxygen or (2) halothane, nitrous oxide + oxygen or (3) thiopentone, halothane, nitrous oxide + oxygen or (4) P.M. (meperidine + atropine) thiopentone, halothane, nitrous oxide + oxygen	Mean duration for group (1) = 26 min (2) = 30 min (3) = 25 min (4) = 46 min	P.T. then at 15 min intervals until P.T. values were attained	No statistically significant differences were noted between the recovery of the groups. All were judged to be fully recovered after 90 min
1965	Vickers	See earlier			See earlier			No tests of statistical significance were employed in this study, but CFF thresholds were found to be depressed for a long time after thiopentone
1980	Wernberg *et al.*	See earlier						Significant changes with 20% and 30%
1984	Azar *et al.*	See earlier			See earlier			Patients from all three treatment groups demonstrated impaired performance at the 1 h test, but all had regained their P.T. performances by the 2 h test

156

Year	Author			N	Age	Patients	Anaesthetic			Results
1979	Gelfman et al.	See earlier		See earlier	See earlier					The groups all showed a significant improvement over the test period indicating a practice effect. Performance was impaired at the immediate postoperative test in both experimental groups
1969	James	See earlier		See earlier	See earlier					The control group showed a significant improvement on the second postoperative day. The experimental group were significantly impaired when compared to the control group on the first postoperative day and did not show the same improvement as the control group on the second day
Coin counting test										
1984	Antonios et al.	50		17–55 mean = 33	Patients undergoing minor gynaecological surgery	Either (1) alfentanil (8 μg/kg), etomidate (0.3 mg/kg), nitrous oxide + oxygen or (2) etomidate (0.3 mg/kg), nitrous oxide + oxygen	Group (1) 8.1 min and group (2) 99 min	P.T. then repeated every 2 min until the P.T. values were obtained	The halothane group required significantly longer than the alfentanil group to attain their P.T. performance

157

Date	Authors	Number of subjects	Age (years)	Population type	Anaesthetic treatment and dosages	Duration of anaesthesia	Test times	Test results
1976	Gale	See earlier			See earlier			The control group's results were unaffected by practice. The long halothane group showed the greatest impairment lasting over the 90 min test. Diazepam also affected performance until 50–70 min test. Methohexitone produced impairment lasting over the 25–50 min test, but the short halothane group were recovered by this time
1965	Vickers	See earlier			See earlier			The test was found to be rather unreliable with marked changes in the results of the same subject (without drugs) on repeated testing. Impairment was found to be greatest following the higher doses of thiopentone and methohexitone and least with the low dose of methohexitone

158

Tests of vigilance 1985 Anderson *et al.*	See earlier	See earlier	Patients in the hyoscine group were significantly slower to complete the test and made more errors than those in the atropine and placebo groups 1 h after surgery. In the last trial (3 h) the hyoscine group were still significantly slower than the placebo group
1984 Antonios *et al.*	See earlier	See earlier	Both experimental groups completed significantly fewer lines at both the 30 and 60 min tests, but there were no differences between the groups. The number of errors per line was significantly greater in the halothane group than in the alfentanil group at both times

159

Date	Authors	Number of subjects	Age (years)	Population type	Anaesthetic treatment and dosages	Duration of anaesthesia	Test times	Test results
Deletion of 'P's and perceptual speed tasks								
1983	Cooper et al.	See earlier	See earlier		See earlier			Patients who received the middle dose of alfentanil produced significantly more errors than all other groups. No other statistically significant differences were observed in either the error score or the number of lines completed
1973	Dixon and Thornton	See earlier			See earlier			The control group showed a significant improvement over the test sessions in speed and accuracy. Patients who received diazepam and local anaesthetic showed a significant decrease in speed immediately after surgery
1981	Edwards et al.	See earlier			See earlier			A significant reduction in scores was observed for 6 days following surgery

| 1979 | Gelfman *et al.* | See earlier | See earlier | The control group showed no improvement with practice. Both experimental groups demonstrated a significant decrease in their performance for over 3 h following surgery. No significant differences were observed between the two experimental groups |
| 1980 | Gelfman *et al.* | See earlier | See earlier | No practice effects were observed in the control group. Both drug combinations produced significant postoperative impairment immediately and 3 h following surgery. The group who received fentanyl were significantly more impaired than the no fentanyl group at the immediate postoperative test |

Date	Authors	Number of subjects	Age (years)	Population type	Anaesthetic treatment and dosages	Duration of anaesthesia	Test times	Test results
1983	Hovorka et al.	See earlier	See earlier		See earlier			1 h and 2 h after their operation, the fentanyl group were significantly more impaired than the enflurane group. Both groups were impaired following surgery but had regained their P.T. scores by the 3 h test
1976	Korttila	See earlier	See earlier		See earlier			No significant changes were observed following diazepam
1983	Riis et al.	See earlier	See earlier		See earlier			Two days after surgery, the groups who received general anaesthesia. General anaesthesia with epidural showed significantly more impairment than the epidural group
1960	Robson et al.	See earlier	See earlier		See earlier			Following nitrous oxide, subjects performed only 62% as well as their pretreatment performances

1971	Rollason *et al.*	See earlier	See earlier	With the scores of all tests ranked and combined, no differences were observed between the groups. Details are not given of the deletion of 'p's test alone
1983	Sinclair and Cooper	See earlier	See earlier	Significantly fewer lines were completed following surgery in both groups. No significant differences were observed in the error scores, when the experimental groups were compared
1964	Eckenhoff *et al.*	See earlier	See earlier	No significant post-operative changes were observed between the groups
1972	Blenkarn *et al.*	See earlier	See earlier	No differences were observed between the two experimental conditions following anaesthesia

163

Physiological assessments
Electroencephalograph recording (EEG)

Date	Authors	Number of subjects	Age (years)	Population type	Anaesthetic treatment and dosages	Duration of anaesthesia	Test times	Test results
1966	Doenicke et al.	38 (each subject used approx. 4 times)		Healthy volunteers	Either (1) thiopentone or thiobutobarbitone (1,000,500 or 250 mg) or (2) methohexitone (150 mg) or (3) propanidid (500 mg) or (4) droperidol peridol (25 mg) + fentanyl (0.5 mg) or (5 dehydrobenzperidol (25 mg) (alcohol also given with some)		Up to 24 h after sedation	The effects of propanidid rapidly diminished, but this did not occur with other agents. After 12 h the effects of methohexitone, thiopentone + thiobutobarbitone, when given with alcohol, were still discernible
1967	Doenicke et al.	See earlier			See earlier			EEG records indicated that fitness was reduced for up to 8 h following barbiturate or ether anaesthesia. Propanidid produced initial impairment but this only lasted 30 min

Maddox Wing

Year	Author	No.	Age	Patients	Method	Recovery	Test	Results
1970	Hannington-Kiff	65	55–64 (in 10 yr age groups)	Dental out-patients	Either (1) 1% methohexitone (1.2 mg/kg) (2) 2.5% propanidid (4.0 mg/kg) (3) 2.5% thiopentone (3.6 mg/kg) These groups also received nitrous oxide + oxygen (and some also had halothane). (4) received nitrous oxide + oxygen with halothane (1–2%)	3–11 min, but most less than 5 min	P.T. then every 5 min for 30 min	The halothane groups show the fastest recovery, followed by the methohexitone and propanidid groups. The thiopentone patients were the worst at the 30 min test, with only 30% of the patients in this group not showing postoperative extra-ocular imbalance
1972	Hannington-Kiff	57	10–59 (in 10 yr age groups)	Minor surgical outpatients	Either (1) Althesin (0.05 ml/kg) or (2) methohexitone (1.2 mg/kg); maintained in both groups by nitrous oxide + oxygen	Group (1) = 4.8 min group (2) = 3.1 min	P.T. 10 min + 30 min after injection	10 min after treatment the divergence from P.T. scores was significantly greater in group 2.

Aspects of Recovery from Anaesthesia: Issues and Comments

I. Hindmarch, J. G. Jones and E. Moss

In writing this overview of the verbal exchange which followed the oral presentation of the previous papers we are giving our understanding of the comments, issues, opinions, criticisms and ideas raised in debate.

An important caveat is that the effects of anaesthetics and analgesics are governed by the dose regimen which is employed and that there exists a great inter-patient variability in response to the various agents. Furthermore, differences in surgical technique, the sex and age of the patients, the timing, nature and method of psychometric assessment and the local hospital conditions will all affect the results of post-operative measures of psychological function and cognitive ability. Such caveats and considerations do not preclude the validity of many of the generalizations made in the précis which follows.

Organization of Day Case Surgery

Although the best way to organize day case surgery is, evidently, in a dedicated day case unit where the whole system is geared to this type of surgery, there are no principles or differences in management which prevent it being done from an in-patient surgical ward. The absence of a day-case unit does not preclude day case surgery. It is also possible to have a separate day case surgical unit provided that patients can be admitted to an acute unit if they are unfit to go home or experience complications.

Age

Children are ideal patients for day case operations, but it is debatable as to whether intravenous or inhalational induction of anaesthesia is more satisfactory; although recovery characteristics are a little better after inhalation compared with intravenous induction of anaesthesia in children. Old age alone is not a contraindication to day case surgery because patients must be assessed individually. The selection is based on their physical status and home circumstances.

Post-operative Analgesia

From the patient's point of view post-operative pain is one of the most frightening features of day case surgery and, therefore, post-operative analgesia is one of the greatest problems with day cases. Local analgesia is useful but oral analgesics are required when the local analgesic wears off. There is considerable individual variation in requirements but for patients undergoing, for example, hernia repair as day cases, the average consumption is five pethidine and 15 Distalgesic tablets. Parenteral non-steroidal anti-inflammatory agents such as nefopam and diclofenac are also useful in day case surgery.

Following cystoscopy, many patients complain of a 'burning sensation' for about 24 hours which can be ameliorated using bupivacaine instilled into the bladder. Such procedures might be unnecessary after cystoscopy alone but following diathermy the post-operative discomfort is much worse and instillation of local analgesic may be helpful.

Consent for Day Case Surgery and Anaesthesia

A special consent form for day case surgery is advisable so that it can be proved that the patients have been given certain accepted instructions before anaesthesia. Before having a general anaesthetic, day case patients should give written confirmation that they have fasted for the required time, made arrangements to be accompanied home and that they will not be alone, drink alcohol, drive a car, operate machinery, use a cooker, or look after small children for 24 hours after their anaesthetic.

Sore Throat

The incidence of sore throat following nasotracheal anaesthesia with packing of the pharynx can be reduced by using dry vaginal tampons. The incidence of sore throat following an anaesthetic using a mask and airway is probably due to the airway and the inhalation of dry anaesthetic gases. The heightened incidence of sore throat after packing the pharynx is still a problem and no particular method of packing has convincingly been proven to reduce the incidence or severity of sore throat.

Pre-operative Medication for Day Cases

Premedication is sometimes required for very anxious people presenting for day case surgery. Temazepam, because of its short duration of action, is accepted as the most suitable of the available benzodiazepines but oral midazolam would probably be equally effective. Midazolam is very short acting and does not give much latitude with the timing of administration.

Benzodiazepine Antagonists

Although benzodiazepine antagonists may be useful in the treatment of benzodiazepine overdose, there does not seem to be an obvious place for using them routinely in day case anaesthesia.

Vomiting after Etomidate

Patients anaesthetized with etomidate have vomited more than those who had received methohexitone or Althesin although the use of droperidol has reduced the incidence of vomiting.

Comparison of Potency of Intravenous Anaesthetic Agents

There is a basic difficulty in quantifying the potency of different anaesthetic agents. Some researchers judge the intensity of effect of intravenous agents by measuring the degree of depression of the median EEG frequency whereas others use power spectral edge and evoked responses for assessing the depth of anaesthesia. The power spectral edge technique is very good at detecting the onset of anaesthesia but on recovery from anaesthesia the patient is wide awake with the spectral edge indicating that the patient is still anaesthetized. The median EEG frequency is a little better, but most EEG based techniques are very prone to artefact and to errors in interpretation.

At present there is no reliable method of measuring the potency of individual drugs so it is impossible to compare accurately the relative potencies of different drugs. It seems that the only method of obtaining some measure of equipotency is to observe the effects of the drug in patients. Anaesthetists will, doubtlessly, choose anaesthetic agents which 'work' and a clinical comparison of potency can, therefore, be obtained from a consideration of the dose regimen of different agents which produce similar conditions of anaesthesia. The overriding difficulty in determining equipotency remains the considerable inter-patient variability in the doses of drugs required to produce the same depth of anaesthesia.

Dreaming following Alfentanil/Propofol Anaesthesia

The evidence regarding dreaming following a combination of alfentanil and propofol remains equivocal. Vivid but not unpleasant dreams during day case anaesthesia with alfentanil and propofol are sometimes reported but equally not mentioned even though there is ample opportunity (on questionnaires) to record such experiences.

Tests of Psychological Functioning

It would appear that many tests of psychological activity relate to 'artificial situations' in laboratories devoid of real life relevance. However, well-validated and reliable psychometric assessments have been shown to reflect the situation of post-operative patients in vehicle handling and in coping with the cognitive demands of daily living.

The practicalities of measuring post-anaesthesia patients necessitates a strict adherence to principles of experimental design and methodology as it is too easy, because of insensitive measures and poor study design, to *fail* to detect the residual effects of anaesthetic agents and therefore to assume, quite wrongly, that such agents are *without* any residual activity on psychological function.

A proper regard of current theory and experimentation is most necessary when 'memory' function is to be measured. There are many modalities of memory. Anaesthetics and 'pre-meds' have a different and often diffuse effect on the various aspects of memory—effects which are often difficult to determine unless a due and proper regard is made of theories and techniques for investigating information processing.

Anaesthetists and psychologists looking for tests of cognitive function should use only those measures which have been shown to be sensitive to the effects of psychoactive drugs and only those which have a proven reliability in use.

Differences between results obtained with the same measure and same anaesthetic used on different occasions are more often due to protocol variations and differences in methodology and experimental design than to any basic differences in the substance under investigation. It is imperative that studies of post-operative recovery of psychological function allow sufficient time for adequate pre-operative baselines to be established. Such baselines, essential for control and analysis of all experiments, can only be obtained *after* the patients have had adequate training and experience of the test measures.

Even with adequate experimental designs and sensitive, reliable and valid measures there still remains the problem of what criterion to use when deciding a patient is 'fit to return home'. It would seem impossible to decide, unlike determining an illegal level of blood alcohol, what objective measure would be used to characterize an unacceptable level of psychological function. Perhaps it is simply necessary to identify those agents that produce residual effects and differentiate them from those which do not produce such disruptive activity. Then, other things being equal (clinical equipotency, ease of administration, cost, interaction with other or adjuvant medications) a list of anaesthetic agents suitable for day case surgery could be drawn up to guide those anaesthetists working with patients who have quickly to return to their habitual ambulatory day-time activities.

Index